The Healing Power of Sleep

By

Marcus J. Gill

&

Fernando Sindaco

Foreward by Dr. Candace Esposito

Disclaimers:

Medical disclaimer

This book is not intended as a substitute for the medical advice of physicians. The reader should regularly consult a physician in matters relating to his/her health and particularly with respect to any symptoms that may require diagnosis or medical attention

Contents:

Sleep Assessment: 9

Introduction: 21

Section 1: 25

    The Great Mystery – What is Sleep? 25

        How did the subservience of sleep happen? 28

    The 5 Sleep Cycles 32

    How does sleep affect us? 36

    Pulling Back the Covers on Sleep 36

        Taking out the Trash 36

        Sleep and Memory 39

        Sleep and Immune Memory 40

        Sleep and Hormones 42

The Problem with Insomnia – it's not
what you think 43

Dreams 45

Pain and Sleep 47

Section 2: Sleep Hygiene 51

What is Sleep Hygiene? 51

Light 52

Noise 56

Temperature 62

Lifestyle 62

Compartmentalized 66

Tips for good sleep hygiene: 68

Section 3: The Sleep System 71

What is a Sleep System? 71

Goldilocks in the bedroom 72

Sleep System in a nutshell: 72

Support 73

Pressure relief 74

Temperature regulation 74

Motion transfer..75

Section 4: Putting the Sleep Myths to Bed 77

Myth No. 1: We all need 8 hours sleep a night 77

Myth No. 2: Sleeping pills help you sleep 82

Myth No. 3: There's an epidemic of sleep
deprivation and we are getting less sleep than
we used to 85

Section 5: The Spiritual Aspect of Sleep 91

New Age meets Ancient Egypt in Dreams.............100

Hypnosis and Dream Cures.......................................103

Shamanism and Schizophrenia 103

The Cult of the Individual 108

Lucid Dreaming 112

Hypnagogic naps 115

The Elephant in the Room

The elephant represents the deep, beautiful, tragic and intelligent mystery of sleep. Elephants as a species are huge and dangerous to any one person, but when respected for what they are and the gifts they bring to us, we would allow ourselves the beauty and wonder that they bring. The same can be said for Sleep. It is mysterious, dangerous if not respected, and beautiful.

Sleep has become the elephant in the room - the big issue everyone is at least vaguely aware of, but tries to ignore, sidestep or downgrade. Why? Because apparently "Sleep is for the weak" and it's become a matter of pride and a badge of honor for some to boast they can get by on four hours a night.

Our mission is to show you that sleep is the gateway to our own inner mysteries and our outer success. The cover represents the beauty and mystery that we can experience when we make deep restorative sleep an everyday sacred ritual.

On another plane, sleep is the ever present leveler of men, without which the king and the pauper alike cannot thrive. Despite its importance and the huge space sleep occupies in our lives, sleep is the first thing we are willing to sacrifice when we have other "stuff" to do. We take sleep for granted, expecting it to serve us and make our lives work but too few are willing to pay sleep's dues.

Sleep is a symptom of caffeine deprivation. ~ANONYMOUS

Sleep Assessment:

	Y	N
Do you wake up without an alarm clock?		
Do you wake up feeling refreshed?		
Do you need caffeine to jump start your day?		
Do you fall asleep quickly?		
Do you wake up in the night and go back to sleep easily?		
Do you find going to sleep difficult?		
Do you have sleep apnea?		
Do you snore?		
Do you suffer from restless legs?		
Do you suffer from nightmares?		
Do you finish your last meal 3 hours before going to bed?		
Is your bedroom dark?		
Do you sleep with your cell phone close by?		
Is your thermostat set below 69°F?		
Would you call yourself a restless sleeper?		
Do you sleep longer over the weekends than on weekdays?		
Do you have at least one hour between screen time and bedtime?		

Do you get up multiple times a night to go to the bathroom?		
Do you wear blue blocking glasses at night?		
Do you work in your bedroom at night before sleep?		
Do you have a bed time ritual where you prepare for sleep?		
Do you work/watch T.V./read on a device in bed?		
Do you rate the quality of your sleep overall as good?		
Do you exercise more than 3 times a week?		
Do you need to take a sleeping pill to get to sleep?		
Do you think you need more sleep?		
Are you irritable a lot of the time?		
Are you impulsive?		
Do you take risks when driving?		
Is the stress in your life under control?		
Do you switch on the light at night to go to the bathroom?		
Are you somewhat forgetful?		
Are you feeling unfocused?		
Are you clumsier than you used to be?		
Do you crave carbohydrates?		
Are you still feeling perky at 11 am and 2 pm?		

Marcus J. Gill would like to acknowledge:

Milcah Ray Josh Feinberg & Scott Davis and the corporate office team for creating a life changing Sunday morning experience

Erik Trammel: For your contagious intensity and passion for carrying out the mission of giving people great sleep.

James Singley: For reminding us to stop apologizing for being who I am and to step up,embrace it and share my best self with the world

Jason Long: For believing in me and giving me an opportunity to reach my full potential and pairing me up with Sidney Williams

Jay Wilson: For his unapologetic authentic drive to win

Michael Alston: Being a great motivator when things look grim

Sidney Williams: True Sleep/bedding expert, mentor and above all friend

Jordan Johnson: For showing me what it looks like to cut through the b.s. in life.

Montana Gangwer for constantly sharing best practices on helping guests get a great night sleep

Tony Young for inspiring me to think past my own selfish ambition

Tracy Ly for making me feel safe to give my all and "drink the kool aide"

Daisy Hernandez for positive energy you bring to our group

Dominique Triston for showing me how to persevere during personal difficulties

Chris Bradshaw for showing me how to change people's lives

with the adjustable bases

Brent McNeil for being an overall good friend and confidant

Garland Smith for making me feel welcome into this great industry

Gary Trentham for takng the time to share best practices and encourage me to be my best

Russell Thompson for sharing his passion and clarity during our training.

Cody Kelly for sharing his expertise and just being a great friend.

Brittany Rankin for showing all amateurs how running a business is really done

Cody Kemp for always being a go to resource for sound business advice

James Gamez my brother from another mother. We've had a good run and I'm looking forward to many more years of bucking the system

Anna Barba Poindexter: For sacrificing everything to give us a better life.

Natana Gill: For Always introducing me to the cool stuff in life.

Cassandra Gaudet: For providing a foundation that allows us to grow.

My little Z: You will always be daddy's baby girl.

Nicole Miles: For being an awesome friend and na.

Alejandro Barba: So proud of you bro! And look forward to helping you with your first book.

Fernando Sindaco: For jumping into this project with both fee

Fernando's Acknowledgments:

I would like to take this time to dedicate this body of work to my mother Martha Bressan who has given me the reason for living the good life. This is for you.

There are so many people I have to thank for the inspiration for this work I hope I don't miss anyone.

Thank you to Garland Smith for seeing something in me that I didn't see in myself

Tony Young for teaching me how to bring people value.

Jocelyn Ruiz for giving me honest feedback

Marcus Gill for putting up with me during this project

Montana Gangwer for being a great friend and a source of inspiration

Brent McNeile for always helping me be more creative

Russell Thompson for always being supportive

Chris Bradshaw for always being a great feedback partner

Amir Baha, for teaching me the value of self-education and teaching me how to sell.

Laura Tscheiller Bressan for being an amazing big sister. Without her, I wouldn't be here today. Thank you for protecting me when I couldn't protect myself.

Valeria Sindaco for being an amazing cousin and a wonderful human being. We are both cut from the same cloth and for that, I am truly grateful.

Eduardo Sindaco my brother and blood. Thanks for showing me what discipline and strength are all about and how to use those qualities in life.

Jason Long for always being a pillar of ethics and trusting me to be creative on your team.

Grant Cardone for being my uncle G, who always pushes me to think bigger and take my actions to 10 X levels.

Jeremy Hicks for being like a brother to me and inspiring me daily.

Jose Ramirez for being loyal through the years and for the great photography on this project.

Scott Davis for being genuinely supportive and encouraging through this journey.

Dominique Seraphine for being a source of inspiration and a pillar of confidence.

Kellie Cooper for always following your dreams. You inspire me every day and make me want to keep my dreams alive. I love you girl!

Luiz Dentinho, my jiu-jitsu professor, for helping to sculpt my mind body and emotions to win at life, for that I am deeply grateful.

Chandra Brey for always being a beam of sunshine everywhere you go. That is super inspiring!

Lamar Bailey, my first true love, who always follows her passion and dreams. I would be half the man I am today without knowing you. Thank you!

Bennchoumy Elien. Where do I even begin to express how much impact Ben has had on my life over the years? You are more than a brother to me and a source of constant inspiration.

Zack Foody, for showing me that great things can come out of Brooklyn NY, and that resourcefulness is the ultimate resource

Brittany Rankin for teaching me that sweetness and kindness are a strength. Thank you!

Elizabeth Bajo, for always looking for deeper truth and enlightenment. Your hunger to understand the world and life is inspiring.

Alan Gongora, for always being a great friend and also an inspiring reminder that where we come from doesn't determine who we become.

Clayton Haley for showing me how education and intelligence can change your financial situation when applied with action.

Stephen Blaschke and John Cash Carpenter for being two of the most creative imaginative people I have ever met.

Jerome Sam for being a brother to me and always finding the humor in life.

Jesus Mendez for always inspiring me to think bigger and to never think small.

Manuel Holguin for showing the ways of spirituality and how important a relationship with God is.

Marlon Vidal, who is the funniest person I have ever met in my life. You always amaze me with your shenanigans.

Foreward

What happens when you type in the words "why am I" into Google?

Did you notice the first suggestion Google's autocomplete function (based on the most common searches) offers you to complete that thought is "why am I so tired?"

That says it all.

In five simple words.

An undeniable reflection of our sleep deprived modern society.

You, me, your family, your friends, co-workers... not one of us is invulnerable to poor sleep. No matter who you are, where you live, where you're at in your life... we all share the common, basic need for good sleep.

Fortunately we're living in the golden age of sleep science. Although still largely a mystery, we know more about sleep than ever before.

We know that sleep is when growth hormone is released so that your body can maintain healthy weight and repair muscle damage. Sleep helps to consolidate your memory and literally changes the cellular structure of your brain by providing a wash of cerebral spinal fluid that removes damaging molecules associated with neurodegeneration (the underlying process involved in conditions like Alzheimer's disease and dementia).

When your sleep suffers your level of cortisol, a key stress hormone, is higher – and that makes you eat more and store belly fat. Your thyroid slows down. Insulin doesn't work as well and your blood sugar goes out of balance. Your risk of cancer can even quadruple depending on the severity of your sleep debt. Poor sleep increases your risk of diabetes, metabolic syndrome, and heart disease.

Yet, even knowing all this, when's the last time your doctor asked you about the quality of your sleep?

Perhaps you're thinking, "Okay, Dr. Candice – how about I just take the Ambien my doctor prescribed me and call you in the morning." Pharmaceuticals aren't the answer though. Marcus and Fernando explore the multiple reasons why, doing an excellent job of outlining the solid evidence proving the ineffectiveness of sleeping pills.

Simply put, popping a prescription isn't the solution because poor sleep isn't caused solely by one factor.

We need a broader-based solution. A holistic system.

And that's where The Healing Power of Sleep comes in.

When you improve your sleep by using the system outlined in this book you'll likely experience the following benefits:

- ➢ Better skin health and a more youthful appearance

- ➢ Better emotional balance and relationships

- ➢ Decreased risk of stroke and cardiovascular disease

- ➢ Fewer accidents

- ➢ Lower levels of inflammation

- ➢ Enhanced function of your immune system and lower risk of cancer and infection

- ➢ Hormonal balance

- ➢ Faster rate of weight loss

- ➢ Decreased pain

- ➢ Stronger bones

- ➢ Lower risk of Alzheimer's disease and cognitive decline; better memory

- ➢ Longevity, slower aging

➢ Improved energy

Along with informing ourselves of the science of sleep, we're also in desperate need of absorbing sleep's mystery. I believe that's my favourite part in The Healing Power of Sleep – the reminder of the glorious gift we have access to each and every night through sleep. The stillness that's available to us that comes from a place deeper and more ancient than the unending busyness and noise that surrounds us in our waking lives.

I encourage you to transform your sleep with the help of Marcus, Fernando and The Healing Power of Sleep. While you're at it, you'll also be transforming your health, and your life.

And... you can leave the Google searches for funny cat videos.

Here's to returning from your nightly journey restored, with fresh eyes and a reinvigorated spirit.

Candice Esposito, ND

Founder of the Calm Living Blueprint

Emerald Park, Saskatchewan, Canada

Introduction:

"Sleep is the golden chain that ties health and our bodies together." ~Thomas Dekker (16th century Elizabethan poet)

Remember Chernobyl, Three Mile Island, the Space Shuttle Challenger and the grounding of the Exxon Valdez? These are among the worst man-made and environmental disasters and all have been linked to human error caused by sleep deprivation. 98,000 people die annually in American hospitals due to medical errors. Impossibly long shifts and vanishingly little sleep is practically a rite of passage among doctors. It's not a long stretch to assume that many of these errors can be traced back to fuddled thinking caused by not enough sleep.

This book is designed to do one thing and one thing only: Change your life through teaching you how to achieve the best sleep. We believe that you should not be building sleep into your life, but rather you should build your life around sound quality sleep. Whether you recognize it or not, sleep is the foundation upon which your entire life rests. It is the only single activity that demands so much of our time. Whatever is going on in the rest of your life, you can be sure that sleep shapes it in one way or another. If your sleep is good, it makes everything else better but if your sleep is bad, it makes everything else worse.

Sleep, or lack thereof, affects us physically, mentally, emotionally, sexually and spiritually. It even influences our relationships, careers, decision-making abilities and the likelihood of having or causing an accident. If you are chronically sleep-deprived, no matter how much you exercise or attend to your diet, you increase the risk of developing cancer, dementia, autoimmune conditions, obesity, diabetes, infertility, depression, mental illness, heart disease and a whole slew of other unpleasant outcomes like premature aging. Sufficient, quality sleep is probably the most underestimated path to good health.

The authors of a study published in 2015, *Behaviorally Assessed Sleep* and *Susceptibility* to the *Common Cold*, used objective measures to track 164 people and their sleep practices. Habitually getting six or less hours of sleep every night translated to a four-fold increase in the odds of catching a cold after exposure to the virus over those who got more sleep. Aric Prather, the lead author of the study and assistant professor of psychiatry at UCSF, said, "Short sleep was more important than any other factor in predicting subjects' likelihood of catching cold," He added, "It didn't matter how old people were, their stress levels, their race, education or income. It didn't matter if they were a smoker. With all those things taken into account, statistically sleep still carried the day." [14]

You may be thinking, so what? Catching the odd cold is not really something to worry about, so this study might seem to be insignificant. However, what the study highlights is that routine sleep deprivation results in low-grade inflammation, confirmed by other studies that show missing out on sleep sets pro-inflammatory processes in motion.

Inflammation can either be your friend or your enemy. Acute inflammation is an emergency reaction and the body's natural and necessary short term response to shock and injury. It is usually visible and dramatic, like the swelling, redness and pain at the site of an injury.

Chronic or low-grade inflammation, on the other hand, is silent and much more subtle. This type of inflammation is not helpful or healing and is, in fact, associated with every so called disease of civilization, some of which were mentioned above – cancer, dementia, autoimmune conditions, obesity, diabetes, depression and heart disease.

Now, the obvious and simple answer to our ills would be to sleep more, right? Unfortunately, as we all know, simple is very seldom easy and this applies to sleep as

[14] http://www.medicalnewstoday.com/articles/298785.php

much as it does to anything else. Most people would love to just sleep more and the reasons why they can't or don't are not simple. To unpack these reasons, we first have to define what sleep is, what it really means and why it is so important. We also have to delve into the importance of getting good sleep rather than just getting more sleep.

What you learn in the following pages may surprise you as you discover the true significance of spending time in the land of nod.

> *"[S]leep deprivation is an illegal torture method outlawed by the Geneva Convention and international courts, but most of us do it to ourselves." ~Ryan Hurd, Dream Like A Boss, 2014*

Section 1:

The Great Mystery – What is Sleep?

The short answer to this question is–we don't know. You can expect to spend roughly a third of your life asleep and if you reach the age of 70 years, some 21 to 25 of them would have been filled with sleep. Despite having to devote this enormous chunk of our lives to sleep, we don't really know what it is. Author David K. Randall calls this state of ignorance "one of the dirty little secrets of science".

Of course, we all know that we need sleep because when we attempt to go without it for an extended period of time, the consequences aren't pretty. We can also describe what happens during sleep – the eyes close, the muscles and nervous system quiet down, the person becomes unresponsive to outside stimuli and their consciousness appears to become suspended. We can even describe what happens to our brain waves during sleep and predict when dreams are likely to occur but we still do not completely understand what this thing called sleep actually is.

Part of that is because sleep is subjective and so very different from our waking lives and so we struggle to define it when we use the state of wakefulness as the template for what is real and valid in experience and only describe sleep in contrast to it.

> *"The great modification which the act of awakening effects in us is not so much that of ushering us into the clear life of consciousness, as that of making us lose all memory of the slightly more diffused light in which our mind had been resting, as in the opaline depths of the sea. The tide of thought, half veiled from our perception, on which we were still drifting a moment ago, kept us in a state of motion perfectly sufficient to enable us to refer to it by the name of wakefulness. But then our actual awakenings produce an interruption of memory. A little later we describe these states as sleep because we no longer remember them." ~Marcel Proust, The Guermantes Way*

What if we are looking at it sleep in the wrong way altogether? Allan Rechtschaffen, sleep researcher at the University of Chicago, said "If sleep doesn't serve an absolutely vital function, it is the greatest mistake evolution ever made." In other words, sleep must have evolved for a very good reason but we are still trying to figure it out.

In an explosion of sleep science over the past 50 years, researchers have been feverishly searching for that 'vital function' and asking exactly what sleep is for. The quest however, almost always involves how sleep benefits wakefulness. What if sleep was more than just a servant to our waking lives?

Sleep and dream specialist Dr. Ruben Naiman says, "Most research looks at sleep and asks questions like how we use sleep to help us perform better. How it will help us improve our immunity? How it will help us be more alert? How it will help us increase our creativity? These are all very important questions but they all presume that sleep is simply in service of the waking. So that way we end up trying to circumvent it. There is a lot of research now going into waking pills. How can we get by without sleep?"

He goes on to say that "We need to remember that sleep, in addition to providing all the service to waking life, is an event in and of itself. Sleep delivers something. It takes us to another place of When we recognize that, we really shift our attitudes towards sleep as something we can actually enjoy not something we simply need to do to be healthier." [2]

How did the subservience of sleep happen?

Sleep belongs to the spiritual, intuitive, nonphysical domain that is not governed by the language and logic we tend to apply to the waking part of our lives. In the west, this type of dichotomy exists everywhere, from education to vocation and how we tend to judge other people. The arts, intuition, music and spirituality are considered the nice-to-have but unimportant parts of life whilst anything to do with mathematics, medicine, science, productivity and work is viewed as the real deal. Of course we use language to propagate these ideas and we are obsessed with naming, labelling, pigeonholing, measuring and compartmentalizing *everything*.

This all stems from the fact that we have two hemispheres in the brain connected by a thick cord of nerve fibers called the corpus callosum. Each hemisphere views the world quite differently but the corpus callosum merges these two views into one seamless version, so we don't notice the difference. The left side (governing the right side of the body) uses a verbal, analytical, convergent, exclusive and sequential mode of thinking, similar to

---

[2] http://articles.mercola.com/sites/articles/archive/2010/11/27/dr-naiman-on-sleep.aspx

how a computer works. The right side uses a nonverbal, intuitive, divergent, inclusive, spatial, holistic and parallel (non-sequential) mode. The left is more concrete and the right is more creative.

As language is so important to our Eurocentric worldview, the left hemisphere, which governs the right side of the body, came to be known as the dominant or major side while the right hemisphere was relegated to the subordinate or minor position.

It is no accident that 'right' (governed by the left hemisphere) also means *true, correct* and *proper*, originating from the Old English word *riht*, meaning *good, fair* and *just*. The synonyms for 'left' (governed by the right hemisphere) are *absent, missing* and *discarded*. It comes from the Old English *lyft*, meaning *weak* or *foolish*.

In *Drawing on the right Side of the Brain*, Betty Edwards explains it like this: "Now, it's important to remember that these terms were all made up, when languages began, by some persons' left hemispheres–the left brain calling the right bad names! And the right brain–labelled, pinpointed and buttonholed–was without a language of its own to defend itself."

All of this goes a long way to explaining why we don't take sleep as seriously as we should. If doctors, scientists and researchers can't explain what sleep is, what chance do we as mere mortals have? We can't pin sleep down, measure it, quantify it, put it in a box or *make* it happen and that flies in the face of our need to structure, rationalize and analyze.

So sleep is the right-brained, non-verbal activity that has been downgraded by the left-brained, verbal waking state. We live in a right-handed world largely dominated by the left brain and this has been the case since the emergence of the ancient civilizations of the Mesopotamians, Egyptians, Greeks and Romans, who all looked down upon left handers, and thus right brainers.

> *"SLEEP - Those little slices of death, how I loathe them." ~Edgar Allen Poe (19th century American poet)*

To the ancient Romans and the Greeks, sleep was pretty much like death, a state hovering between this world and the next. In fact Hypnos, the Greco-Roman god of sleep, was the twin brother of Thanatos, the god of death. They were the sons of the primordial goddess of the night, Nyx, who was the mother of all things mysterious and "anything that was inexplicable, such as death, disease, sleep, ghosts, dreams, witchcraft and enchantments." [3]

The Romans have been described as being in left brain overdrive and they were particularly suspicious of doing anything left handed. Our English word *sinister* comes

---

[3] http://www.talesbeyondbelief.com/greek-gods-mythology/nyx.htm

straight from the Latin for left. Even as late as the mid twentieth century in this country, children were punished for writing with their left hand and Catholic nuns used to declare the left was the hand of the devil.

Over the centuries then, this fear of and disregard for anything that can't be pinned down, explained logically or easily duplicated has seeped into our collective psyche and sleep has been left out in the cold. Most of us sleep not because we want to or because we love to but we because we grudgingly admit that we have to. We are a society that has forgotten we are human beings and not human doings, giving rise to thoughts like this one from Donald Knuth, "The hardest thing is to go to sleep at night, when there are so many urgent things needing to be done."

Keep all this in mind as you read the rest of this book as we try to illuminate the value of something that has been subtly undervalued and discriminated against for centuries–sleep.

"The incomparable respite and rejuvenation offered us in sleep is not a subtraction from but is an enhancement of life." ~Dr. Rubin Naiman in Hush: A Book of Bedtime Contemplations

The 5 Sleep Cycles

Until fairly recently, it was widely accepted in conventional medicine that deep sleep, like death or coma, was a state of unconsciousness. Sleep has often been described as an 'absence' either of consciousness or wakefulness. Dictionary.com defines sleep as "A natural periodic state of rest for the mind and body, in which the eyes usually close and consciousness is completely or partially lost". [4]

Contrast this with the teachings of the ancient Indian philosophy of Hinduism, where deep sleep is described as one of three states of consciousness, the other two being waking and dreaming. Now science has revealed that we are not unconscious at all in sleep and just as the ancient Hindus maintained, we are just in a different state of consciousness.

Sleep is actually an incredibly busy time for the brain. While the body becomes more and more immobile, the brain engages in all sorts of activities.

Sleep occurs in repeating cycles consisting of five stages. Each cycle lasts approximately 90 to 110 minutes and each stage lasts between 5 to 15 minutes. The cycle becomes longer than the one before. On any given night's sleep, you will progress through roughly five of these cycles.

---

[4] http://www.dictionary.com/browse/sleep--over

Stages one to four are referred to as non-REM sleep and the fifth and last stage is REM or rapid eye movement sleep. This is the stage that increases the length of each cycle and the one normally associated with dreaming and the establishment of long-term memory.

Stage 1: Also known as N1 or NREM1 is characterized by drowsiness and is that state between being awake and being asleep where the muscles haven't settled down yet and the eyes might roll around and flutter open and closed. Brain waves shift from the beta waves that dominate conscious attention to the slower but more synchronized alpha. In alpha, you can still be attentive but in a more relaxed and open minded way similar to a trance state. Gradually alpha gives way to theta as the waves become slower still.

Physically, breathing regulates and heart rate slows down. This stage is very light sleep so you can still hear what is going on around you but it is muted and relatively easy to ignore. It is during this short stage you might experience those horrible twitches and jerks that shock you briefly awake because you feel as if you are falling.

Stage 2: Also known as N2 or NREM2, this is the first stage of real sleep. You might still be able to hear sounds but they won't mean anything to you and your muscles will be nicely relaxed and inactive. Brain waves are now mostly in the theta range while sleep spindles and K-complexes make an appearance. Spindles are short fast bursts of electrical brain activity that seem to be involved in refreshing our brains in preparation for learning. They are also thought to preserve sleep by inhibiting sensory input.

Stage 2 makes up the majority of sleep and accounts for about half of the total sleep time for an adult and more for those who are younger. More time is spent here than in any other kind of sleep and a sleeper will visit this stage a number of times throughout the night.

Stage 3 & 4: Also known as NREM3 or N3 and delta sleep. It is considered deep, slow wave sleep. In the past they were separated into two stages but now are often referred to as one and the same stage. This is the deepest sleep and it is very difficult to rouse someone from this stage. If you do manage to wake them up, they will feel groggy and be quite disorientated. Everything from neuronal activity to heart rate and breathing are at their lowest point and some dreaming may occur but it will be fragmented and hard to recall. This is the stage where nightmares, bedwetting, sleep talking and sleep walking may happen.

Stage 5: This is the last stage of sleep, called REM or paradoxical sleep. EEG activity in REM sleep is much like that of waking life but is accompanied by sleep paralysis. This REM atonia is achieved by the brain shutting off the stimulus to the large muscle groups and is nature's way of protecting you from imitating what happens in your dreams in real life.

Brain waves in REM sleep range from theta waves to alpha and possibly even high frequency beta waves which you would expect when someone is engaged in concentrating and complex thought. This stage accounts for about a quarter of normal sleep.

At some point, your temperature bottoms out and then starts to increase, along with cortisol. The REM portion of sleep increases and your body starts preparing itself for the move towards wakefulness and a new day.

Brain waves are sorted into five broad categories. At any one time, all five are present but in varying degrees. Delta waves are associated with deep sleep and the unconscious mind and have the slowest frequency. Blue light in the evening is known to disrupt the production of Delta waves later on in the night.

People who struggle to fall asleep or who wake up during the night might experience "Alpha intrusion sleep disorder" where they are suddenly roused from sleep and feel way more alert than they should be but they aren't quite awake enough to make sense of anything.

The fastest frequency is created by Gamma waves but we don't know a whole lot about them except that they involve the entire brain and accompany pure, altruistic thought and genius. In between these two are Theta (sleep, deep meditation, inspiration and dreaming), Alpha (meditative, resting brain state) and Beta (focused, problem solving state).

How does sleep affect us?

"Sleeping is no mean art: for its sake one must stay awake all day." ~Friedrich Nietzsche

Sleep is a physiological need, like drinking and eating. If you did not or could not sleep, you would first go a little crazy and then you would eventually die. In fact, the very rare brain disease fatal familial or sporadic insomnia is a progressive and currently incurable condition where the inability to sleep results in memory loss, dementia and death.

We know that the persistent myth that the brain simply shuts down during sleep is just that, a myth. The brain is very active in sleep and in some ways it is actually more active than when we are awake. The body might be at rest but the brain never gets to take a break.

Pulling Back the Covers on Sleep

Taking out the Trash

You have probably heard of the lymphatic system, the body's garbage disposal and infection-fighting division. This vital part of the immune system was discovered as far back as the seventeenth century but what had always puzzled scientists is that it did not extend to the brain. It was assumed that the central nervous system (the brain and spinal cord) was an immune-privileged site devoid of lymphatic vessels.

How the brain cleared itself of waste materials however, was a mystery. It was doubly intriguing considering the importance of the brain to survival and the fact that it is inordinately energy hungry relative to its size. The brain weighs in at 2% of our body mass but hogs between a fifth and a quarter of the body's total energy supply. This means a lot more metabolic waste products than any other organ – in one year, the brain generates its own weight in worn out proteins. So where was it all going?

In 2012, this mystery was solved with the stunning discovery of the brain's very own sophisticated and powerful lymphatic system, dubbed the "glymphatic system". Maiken Nedergaard, head of the team responsible for the discovery said, "It's as if the brain has two garbage haulers – a slow one that we've known about, and a fast one that we've just met...Given the high rate of metabolism in the brain, and its exquisite sensitivity, it's not surprising that its mechanisms to rid itself of waste are more specialized and extensive than previously realized". [5]

By now, you are probably wondering what all this has to do with sleep. Well, it turns out that this newly discovered

[5] https://www.urmc.rochester.edu/news/story/3584/scientists-discover-previously-un-known-cleansing-system-in-brain.aspx

system only kicks into high gear when you sleep. Whether you are awake or asleep, the brain is active and needs energy. Researchers speculate that it is this housekeeping that is largely responsible for the energy consumption in sleep. Sleep quite literally cleans and clears the mind. The converse of this is that lack of sleep pollutes the mind.

> *"the restorative nature of sleep appears to be the result of the active clearance of the by-products of neural activity that accumulate during wakefulness."* [6] *~ Maiken Nedergaard, M.D., D.M.Sc.*

Something else happens during sleep that surprised researchers–to expedite the cleanup, the brain changes its structure. The cells in the sleeping brain shrink some 60% to open up the spaces in between and allow the movement of cerebrospinal fluid through the tissues where it can then flush away debris, old cells and toxic build-up. The glymphatic system whisks the trash away and dumps it into the lymphatic system which carries it to the liver for recycling or removal. No prizes for guessing what happens when you skimp on sleep.

Alzheimer's, Parkinson's, ALS and other neurodegenerative diseases all seem to have one thing in common, the

---

[6] https://www.urmc.rochester.edu/news/story/3956/to-sleep-perchance-to-clean.aspx

accumulation of clumps of toxic proteins in the brain that gum up the works and prevent electrical and chemical signaling. In Alzheimer's, these clumps are called amyloid plaques and in Parkinson's they are known as Lewy bodies.

In a research paper entitled Brain Drain, [7] Maiken Nedergaard and Steven A. Goldman note, "Many patients with Alzheimer's experience sleep disturbances long before their dementia becomes apparent. In older individuals, sleep becomes more fragmented and shallow and lasts a shorter time. Epidemiological studies have shown that patients who reported poor sleep in middle age were at greater risk for cognitive decline than control subjects when tested 25 years later." The authors hypothesized that rather than sleep difficulties being just a side effect of dementia, they might be part of the cause.

Whilst pharmaceutical companies are scrambling to develop drugs that would block the pesky protein clusters in neurodegenerative conditions, perhaps sleep is all the therapy we need to treat what have become known as 'dirty brain' diseases.

Sleep and Memory

When we sleep, our brains sift and sort through information, deciding what is useful to keep and what can be discarded and then they use the end product to

---

[7] https://www.ncbi.nlm.nih.gov/pmc/articles/PMC5347443/

consolidate our memories. If you learn something new and then sleep on it shortly after, you are much more likely to remember it better at a later date. Experiments have shown how sleep following learning strengthens memory.

During REM sleep, when we dream, long term memories are established. If you imagine your head was filled with a whole lot of balloons, with each balloon representing a different aspect of your experience, in sleep your brain would collect a bunch of related balloons from the present and the past and tie them up together. Every time you experience something new, the bunch gets rearranged but each balloon can also belong to multiple bunches.

Your brain does not remember specifics however, only gist information. It extracts and abstracts the most important bits and all the new connections and associations help you to unravel problems now and in the future and find creative solutions to them while we sleep. When you are learning a new skill, sleep is just as important as practice in mastering the skill.

Sleep and Immune Memory

Sleep is not only important for psychological memory but physiological memory too, specifically immunological memory. Just as sleep allows the brain to extract gist information from experiences, it allows the immune system to do the same with information from pathogens. Instead of storing the precise details about a virus or bacterium, the immune system gathers just enough fragments (the gist) to produce memory T cells that will help it identify that pathogen again, along with closely related but not identical pathogens.

In this way, the immune system can mount an immediate defense to invaders because it 'remembers' past encounters. Thus sleep makes your immune system more flexible and responsive, giving it a much more nuanced repertoire of action.

Additionally, hormones released during sleep strengthen the communication between the molecules responsible for identifying threats and those that trigger an immune response. [8] You can see how lack of sleep could make everything fuzzy, from your head to your immunity and how sleep sharpens and polishes our lives.

Have you ever noticed that when you get sick, you just want to sleep? You might put that down to being tired because you are sick but the wisdom of the body is a lot more deliberate than that and it appears that sleep is a function of the immune system. When you are sleep deprived, you are much more likely to succumb to infection and when you get sick, your body creates tiredness so that you will sleep and during sleep, it will launch repair work.

---

[8] https://www.eurekalert.org/pub_releases/2015-09/cp-sms092215.php

Healing takes a lot of energy so it makes sense for our bodies to induce sleepiness and divert energy from physical activity to recovery. Researchers studying the simple roundworm recently discovered that cells under stress (i.e. when ill) cause the release of neuropeptides that signal cells in the nervous system to dial activity down. They suspect a similar mechanism is at play in animals and humans. [9]

Sleep and Hormones

During sleep, especially SWS or slow wave sleep (Stage 3), a whole slew of hormones are impacted. Some are released and others are held back, a process which is reversed in sleep deprivation. For instance, the production of HGH (human growth hormone) is maximized in deep sleep. A deficiency in HGH means you will age faster, have a weaker immune system, more fat, and less muscle strength and mass.

Leptin, the satiety hormone that tells you have had enough to eat, is released in spades when you get deep sleep whilst ghrelin, the hunger hormone has the brakes applied. Lack of sleep not only makes you hungry but hungry for carb-rich, high calorie food and also messes up your glucose tolerance so that any food you do eat is not metabolized efficiently, resulting in fat storage.

---

9 https://www.sciencedaily.com/releases/2017/01/170119120217.htm

On top of this, the adrenal stress hormone cortisol becomes elevated, which adds to the deposition of the dreaded and dangerous belly fat and increases the likelihood of diabetes. High cortisol at night means more insulin resistance in the morning and impaired glucose metabolism during the day. Lack of sleep suppresses the parasympathetic nervous system–the one you need for recovery and healing–and activates the sympathetic nervous system, putting you into a state of high alert. It also subdues the release of prolactin, an anti-inflammatory hormone.

The Problem with Insomnia – it's not what you think

Some people do suffer from insomnia but many people who think they are insomniacs are simply suffering from anxiety about insomnia. This is so widespread that the fixation about not sleeping is a separate problem altogether.

"Insomnia is a gross feeder. It will nourish itself on any kind of thinking, including thinking about not thinking." ~ Clifton Fadiman

When it comes to insomnia, we are our own worst enemies. We don't know how to switch off or stop thinking. It's that left brained thing again where we have convinced ourselves that we can conquer sleep by willing ourselves to do it.

Sleep is a bit like happiness in that it is a by-product. Good sleep is the by-product of good habits just as bad sleep is the by-product of bad habits. You can't catch sleep or produce it and you cannot summon it at will. You can't buy it even and you cannot go to sleep. You can go to your bed but you have to wait for sleep to come to you. You can only surrender to sleep and this is where people probably have the most trouble because they are so accustomed to trying to control everything else in their lives.

> *"Turn resolutely to work, to recreation, or in any case to physical exercise till you are so tired you can't help going to sleep, and when you wake up you won't want to worry."*
> *~ B. C. Forbes*

If you have difficulty sleeping, you might have to work on re-educating your body and mind. Lying awake in bed while you toss and turn trains you to associate being awake with being in bed and eventually this becomes your 'normal'. If you are still awake after 20 minutes, do not lie there fretting about not sleeping but get up and go and do something that will distract you and then go back to bed. Rinse and repeat until you fall asleep.

Another trick is to do your best to try and stay awake. This sounds counterintuitive but if falling asleep is a problem and worrying about it isn't solving it, you need to try something different. Attempting to stay awake can get you out of the rut of obsessing about the fact that you are not sleeping.

You must have heard about the thought experiment called "ironic process theory". According to Wikipedia, it "refers to the psychological process whereby deliberate attempts to suppress certain thoughts make them more likely to surface." So, for instance, if I asked you not to think about a pink elephant, the first image that would pop into your head would be a pink elephant. The same happens with sleeplessness where you can't exclude it by thinking about it.

> "If you can't sleep, then get up and do something instead of lying there worrying. It's the worry that gets you, not the lack of sleep." ~ Dale Carnegie

Dreams

As much as you might worry about lack of sleep, there might be a bigger problem for you to worry about and that is lack of dreams. Dreaming gets even less press and attention than sleep does but this may be a huge mistake. Many sleep specialists pay scant attention to dreaming and most of us think they are just these arbitrary and often bizarre hallucinations that seem so real and vivid at the time but are so easily forgotten.

> *"We are such stuff*
> *As dreams are made on, and our little life*
> *Is rounded with a sleep."*
> ~William Shakespeare, The Tempest

It's easy to write dreams off as unimportant until you consider that they might just be misunderstood. According to Dr. Naiman, "Dreaming is essential. In recent years, there's been a lot of research underscoring the fact that dreaming has functions very different from sleep." [10] Dreams seem to be a way for us to work through our emotional and psychological pain. They help us to make sense of our lives and process things without the intervention of our waking consciousness. In a way, dreams expand our notion of reality and provide another level of experience which can be enjoyed for itself as well as enrich our waking lives.

And there's the hitch–so much of our waking lives actively inhibits dreaming. Shaving an hour or two or three off your sleep steals dream time. Waking up too early to an alarm clock instead of allowing yourself to awaken naturally cuts dreams short. Have you ever been rudely

---

[10] http://articles.mercola.com/sites/articles/archive/2014/07/13/sleeping-dreaming.aspx

awakened in the middle of a dream and felt cheated, like getting to the end of a good novel to find the last few pages missing? There's a reason for that feeling.

Prescription and OTC sleeping pills that are anti-cholinergics, like Benadryl, suppress REM sleep and thus dreaming. Most anti-depressants also have a negative effect on REM sleep which leads to less dreams. Naiman refers to all of this as "dream deprivation" which in turn deprives us of the "digestive and assimilating process for information". [11]

He goes on to say, "I think after this information is digested, the process of assimilation shows up metaphorically in the dream, in the images of the dream. The bottom line here is that if you don't dream well, it has a profoundly negative impact on your memory. In a deeper sense, it's as if you stopped growing psychologically. You stopped adding to who you are."

Pain and Sleep

Pain in general and back pain in particular affect a large percentage of the population and entire books have been written about them. Of interest to us is the impact that pain has on sleep and the impact sleep has on pain.

---

[11] http://articles.mercola.com/sites/articles/archive/2014/07/13/sleeping-dreaming.aspx

Beyond the physical impact that pain has on sleep in that it's difficult to fall asleep and stay that way when you are in pain, there's another surprising and often neglected side to pain–the emotional or mental side. What most people do not realize is that to your brain, both physical and emotional pain are essentially the same thing and are processed in the same area of the brain. Unfortunately, in our left-brained society, there's always a pill for that and yet again, sleep becomes a casualty.

It's no secret to the medical community but it may be one to you that opioid pain killers like codeine, oxycodone, morphine and heroin all offer relief from physical as well as emotional distress. Now consider that while Americans represent 5% of the global population, they consume 80% of the global supply of prescription opioids and 99% [12] of a specific and potent pain killer called hydrocodone, also sold under the brand name Vicodin.

What does this suggest about the society that we live in? Either it means that we are in more pain than any other society or it means that we are doing something very wrong. Addiction to prescription opioids has become a problem of epic proportions and has led to a steep rise in heroin addictions because heroin is cheaper and, surprisingly, less potent.

---

[12] http://www.cnbc.com/2016/04/27/americans-consume-almost-all-of-the-global-opioid-supply.html

All of these prescription pain killers may initially cause drowsiness and help people get to sleep but they also cause havoc with natural sleep patterns over time. The sleep you get with these drugs is not the restorative kind you need, much the same as with sleeping pills– in both cases, you sleep but do not experience REM sleep. Additionally, they can cause memory problems, insomnia, nightmares and what is known as twilight sleep, where you have one foot in sleep and another in wakefulness but can't be fully in either. Of course, when you wake up in the morning, although you have 'slept' you don't feel particularly rested.

Roughly 80% of Americans suffer from back pain at some point in their lives. Some pain resolves itself but in some cases it transforms from the acute kind to the lifelong chronic kind because after a few months, the pain pathways can become fixed. Then people get stuck in a never ending loop of pain that keeps reinforcing itself.

Over one hundred million Americans are in chronic pain right now and this has huge repercussions on our society, from the financial burden to the costs of human misery, lack of life quality and lost productivity. Here is the interesting part–according to Dr. Hanscom, an orthopedic surgeon who wrote *Back in Control,* A Surgeons Roadmap Out of Chronic Pain "Actually lack of sleep is more correlated with disability than the actual amount of pain." [13]

---

[13] http://mercola.fileburst.com/PDF/ExpertInterviewTranscripts/Interview-David Hanscom-TakingChargeOfYourChronicPainTreatment.pdf

Dr. Hanscom treated his own long-term chronic pain successfully and now uses a suite of interventions with his patients to address their stress, diet, medication and emotional dysfunction. Ironically, surgery is something that he generally does not recommend. Expressive writing, where you put down all your deep, dark and negative thoughts on paper forms the bedrock of his treatment but nothing is more important than sleep. He acknowledges that most people with chronic pain don't sleep very well and says, "Sleep is number one. The entire project is null and void unless you're sleeping."

> *"Sleep is number one. The entire project is null and void unless you're sleeping." ~Dr. David Hanscom, orthopedic surgeon*

Section 2:

Sleep Hygiene

What is Sleep Hygiene?

Sleep hygiene is a relatively new term that refers to the best practices for getting good sleep. It involves developing better habits and fostering the right environmental and behavioral modifications necessary for getting to sleep easily and staying asleep so that you can wake up feeling refreshed.

It seems ridiculous to pay attention to something that we should be able to do instinctively but we have veered so far away from the natural order of doing things that we need some help. Good sleep hygiene revolves around four main areas: light, noise, temperature and lifestyle/preparation. If we are honest with ourselves, we have to admit that we have developed some very unhealthy ways of approaching all four.

Light

We live in an amazing time where we can turn night into day and day into night with the flip of a switch. No longer are we governed by sunrise and sunset because we have all these artificial light sources to illuminate the darkness. The day that Edison perfected the light bulb, our relationship with sleep was forever changed.

That single invention paved the way for nightlife, shift work, light pollution, the 24-hour day, the global economy, our always 'on' culture and the separation of man from the rhythms of nature that have guided him for millennia. The ensuing disruption of our internal clocks turned sleep into the biggest casualty. Apparently, Edison didn't care about this because he thought sleep was a waste of time. His humble brag was that he never needed more than three or four hours a night. He was known to work a straight 60 hours without sleep but would then have to sleep for 30. He was also known for napping frequently during the day.

Humans, and every other creature on earth, operate according to circadian rhythms and these rhythms are regulated by light. Light is far more than just something to read by, it is a nutrient. Dr. Liberman, author of *Light: Medicine of the Future,* says, "When we speak about health, balance, and physiological regulation, we are referring to the function of the body's major health keepers; the nervous system and the endocrine system. These major control centers of the body are directly stimulated and regulated by light, to an extent far beyond what modern science...has been willing to accept."

During the day, we should be getting a lot of bright natural light and at night, the complete opposite, a lot of darkness. Instead, we work indoors, mostly in offices lit by synthetic light. Then we go home and flood the night with more artificial light and sleep in the glow of an electric alarm clock or street lights. So not only are we starved of real light but we are exposing our eyes to too much light when they crave the dark. No wonder people's bodies are confused. Professor Russell Foster from Oxford University called us "the supremely arrogant species; we feel we can abandon four billion years of evolution and ignore the fact that we have evolved under a light-dark cycle". [14]

The biggest source of blue light is the sun. This might seem like a warning to avoid the sun but blue light isn't all bad news – it depends where it is coming from and when you get it. During the day, blue light from the sun is energizing and helps stave off things like depression. The dark side of blue light is that it triggers the production of reactive oxygen species in our tissues, also known as oxidative stress. Reactive oxygen species are a by-product of inflammation but they also contribute to the progression of inflammatory disorders. Sunlight, however, is full spectrum light, so it carries the regenerative and protective red and near-infrared wavelengths too.

---

[14] http://www.bbc.com/news/health-27286872

Artificial light at night is the wrong light at the wrong time. On top of that, it seems we are biologically primed to absorb blue light through our eyes. Unlike UV light which does not penetrate the eye, blue light travels right to the back of the eye, making us particularly vulnerable to it at night.

> *Top Tip: Go camping! "Scientists at the University of Colorado Boulder found that if you live by the sun's schedule, you are more likely to go to bed at least an hour earlier, wake up an hour earlier, and be less groggy, because your internal clock and external reality are more in sync. The sun adjusts your clock to what may be its natural state, undoing the influence of lightbulbs."*

You might have heard of the sleepy time hormone of darkness, melatonin. It is often used as a sleep aid and although it is very important for sleep, it has many other essential functions in the body. Melatonin is a powerful anti-inflammatory, an antioxidant, a free radical scavenger and an immunomodulator–meaning that it influences the immune system. Melatonin also increases the effects of some antioxidants and protects others from the damage of oxidation. Melatonin helps shield your DNA from harm and has far reaching effects on almost every other hormone in your endocrine system.

Melatonin is thus hugely important but blue light in the evening suppresses it. The millions of people vegging out in front of the television at night are also giving themselves a big dose of blue light too. Due to the nature of the media, watching TV also dilates your pupils. This means you become somewhat hypnotized and unblinking, causing even more light to enter the eyes.

It has been known for some time that breast cancer occurs more frequently in women who are exposed to light at night, for instance those who work shifts or have night jobs. This seems to be tied to melatonin as studies have shown that the lower the levels of the hormone, the faster the growth of the tumor.

Melatonin is mainly secreted by the pineal gland but the retina, lens and iris also produce it. In the eye, it acts as an antioxidant and regenerates the rods and the cones. You can see how blue light would have a negative effect upon eye health and impose a sort of "biological darkness" by disturbing the light/dark cycle and consequently the production of melatonin.

"In mammals, the melatonin rhythm is generated by an endogenous circadian master clock in the suprachiasmatic nucleus (SCN) of the hypothalamus, which is entrained by the light/dark cycle over a 24-hr period." [15]

---

[15] https://www.ncbi.nlm.nih.gov/pmc/articles/PMC3001216/

Noise

When we talk about noise, we don't just mean the type that involves your neighbor's teenage son revving their motorbike at midnight. That is just one type of noise but there are others. Noise stands for interference—anything that distracts you from putting your head down and getting to sleep.

Noise can be grouped into three categories: mind noise, body noise and environmental noise. Too much of any of them can prevent good sleep by putting you into or keeping you stuck in a state of arousal instead of the calm and relaxed state necessary for slumber. As the evening wears on, your sleepiness should increase and the noise levels should decrease.

Mind noise

You are dog tired and you crawl into bed, anticipating that wonderful oblivion called sleep. You lay your head down on the pillow and close your eyes, hoping to drift off to dreamland. Just as you take a leisurely breath in and out, a disturbing thought pops into your head and you start fretting about how you are going to pay that medical bill at the end of the month or finish that presentation in time or pick up the kids, do the groceries and make your dentist appointment all at the same time tomorrow and on and on and on...

> *"A ruffled mind makes a restless pillow."* ~
> *Charlotte Brontë*

I am sure you have all been there, where one worrisome thought leads to another and suddenly, no matter how sleepy you were to start with, you can't sleep for all the thinking. This condition has a charmingly evocative name, it's called cognitive popcorn. Other types of mind noise are things like anxiety, anger, regret and any other negative emotions that you replay in your mind, thus preventing sleep.

Body noise

Body noise comes in all sorts of flavors, from pain to discomfort, cramps, restless legs, headaches, indigestion, backache, reflux and tension. Some people simply do not know how to relax but it's only when they get into bed that they have the time or space to notice how wound up they are and how much everything hurts.

A big part of body noise comes from our sedentary lifestyles and the way we move or fail to move during the day. We sit to eat breakfast, sit in the car/train/bus going to work, sit at a desk all day, sit on the way home and sit some more to eat dinner and watch TV. If this describes your life, you might be exhausted by the time you go to bed, even though you just sat through your day.

There are three problems here. One is that sitting on furniture enables us to stay in one place a lot longer than we should without feeling the need to move. Because the chair or seat is doing the work that our muscles should be doing, we don't notice the lack of circulation or that we are getting stiff. Our bodies are not really designed to sit at the awkward 90° angle of most chairs either, so in the long run, we get back ache and or neck ache.

Two, being sedentary for long stretches of time is extraordinarily unhealthy. It is so bad for us that even going to the gym and exercising every day does not undo the damage. In other words, an hour of exercise is no match for sitting practically motionless all day. That is not to say that exercise is not important, it absolutely is but what may be even more important is simply moving more.

According to Dr. Joan Vernikos, whose job at NASA was to keep astronauts healthy while they were in space, chronic sitting prevents us from pushing against gravity. She says that gravity is our friend but that we age faster when we move less because we are not engaging gravity. Standing instead of sitting all day is not the answer either.

Vernikos says, "Sitting is okay, but it's uninterrupted sitting that is bad for us. We are not designed to sit continuously.... It's not how many hours of sitting that's bad for you; it's how often you interrupt that sitting that is GOOD for you!" Just standing up every 30-40 minutes gets gravity working for you instead of against you.

The third issue is that sitting (along with walking, running, riding a bicycle, climbing stairs and even many of the exercises in a gym) involves one single, overused plane of movement–the sagittal plane. In this plane, we move backwards or forwards but our bodies are also built to move in the frontal (side to side) and transverse (rotational and twisting) planes.

As a result of modern conveniences like cars, escalators and lifts, the older we get, the less we use our bodies. We don't sit on the floor anymore and we don't squat because, hey, we have furniture. In fact, our relationship with the floor gets ever more distant as we get locked into very limited patterns of movement–limited to the car, the chair and the bed and then we blame this on old age.

Muscle imbalances, dysfunctional and restricted ways of moving, muscle injury, pain and, of course, the resultant inability to sleep well are not the automatic consequences of age but of disuse and abuse. As our bodies operate best when they can move through all three planes of motion with ease, the best exercises are functional, whole-body ones that recruit different joints, muscles and planes. In short, we should learn to move like children again and dance, skip, climb, run and crawl. If that seems undignified, there's always Pilates and yoga.

Environmental noise

This includes actual noise like traffic outside your window, a cricket stuck in your bedroom or a snoring partner but also refers to light (covered above) and temperature (covered below). Environmental noise is any interference from the outside world. Perhaps the loudest noise here is simply the way we lead our lives in a fast paced world.

All day long we are exposed to visual and auditory noise from in-your-face advertisements, sirens, music, phones, laptops and televisions. Depending on where you work, you might have to put up with the noise from co-workers, customers or machinery. To keep up, get ahead or just maintain a position, we take stimulants like caffeine or sugar.

> *21st century problem—we are all tired but wired*

In a sense, we are all suffering from sensory overload—we are continually overexcited as if we are stepping on the gas all the time, which leaves us tired but wired. If you are on the go from early in the morning until you finally flop into bed at night without having some sort of transition in between, you are very unlikely to be able to sleep well.

If you engage with other people and or technology all day (podcasts, the radio, computer, smart phone,

Instagram, Facebook, twitter, Skype, Pinterest, television etc.) you are constantly being fed visual and audio distraction and entertainment. The minute your head hits the pillow however, you are confronted with your thoughts and your own unopposed internal dialogue.

This comes part and parcel with treating sleep as something you have to do in order to do the rest of your life better. You have to treat sleep with a little more deference and then sleep will treat you better. That means easing your foot off the pedal and coming down a bit before trying to sleep instead of thinking you can just jump into it.

So how do you create that transition? The trick here is to find something that works for you because one's man's pleasure is another's pain. For instance, some people can unwind when they bake or cook but other people get stressed out at the very thought of getting into the kitchen.

You can meditate, read, write in a journal, take a hot bath, plan your tomorrow, pray, talk to someone, go for a stroll, listen to music–whatever works for you. The goal is to minimize the noise and create a bridge between your waking life and sleep by preparing for and welcoming sleepiness. By the time you get into bed, sleepiness should be elevated and all the noise should be muted so that by the time you wake up in the morning, this can be reversed. This is the real meaning of sleep hygiene.

Temperature

Getting the right temperature at night has a huge influence on sleep. Unfortunately, especially in winter, we tend to think that the warmer, the better. It isn't. To sleep well, the body needs to be on the cool side and being too hot makes sleep very difficult and amounts to a type of environmental noise. Experts recommend setting the thermostat between 60 and 69°.

Another way of looking at temperature is to see that as a society, we are almost always running too hot. We want everything to be bigger, faster, better and we want it now. We constantly push our physical and mental boundaries by burning the metaphorical candle at both ends. This leads to the physical inflammation we talked about earlier but also to a kind of mental inflammation where stress and burn out are the norm rather than the exception.

Lifestyle

If sleep occupies a third of our lives, it seems logical to assume that just about every other thing we do in the other two thirds has some influence on how well we sleep. We have already addressed the importance of getting sufficient natural light during the day but there are a number of other influences like diet and exercise that have a major impact on your quality of sleep.

Exercise

Exercise is the yang to the yin of sleep. You need the exertion of exercise to be able to take full advantage of the peace and rest offered by sleep.

Exercise helps to dissipate stress, increases blood flow, ramps up circulation and gets the lymphatic system pumping, all of which primes your physical and mental states for sleep. One of the best antidotes to depression is to get moving and there is plenty of evidence that exercise is beneficial for insomniacs.

When you do vigorous exercise, you increase your core body temperature and it is thought that the consequent drop in temperature as your body cools down is good for sleep. We have spoken about the fact that we are too hot, too hyped and too frenetic and this is where exercise can disrupt that pattern by providing a safe outlet for arousal and allowing us to decompress.

Any exercise is better than no exercise and even something as simple and free as walking can benefit you. It's a good idea to take up an exercise that you love so that you will keep doing it.

> *Did you know?*
>
> *Tight hamstrings can cause or exacerbate lower back pain which can prevent sleep. Try stretching them daily. An inversion table can also help to decompress and relax the spine.*

Diet

It should come as no surprise that the food you choose to eat can help you sleep better, or not. It works the other way round too because sleep also influences your diet. Sleeplessness leads to cravings for carbs and foods high in sugar and there is an undeniable link between bad sleep and obesity.

The SAD (standard American diet) of highly processed food jam-packed with sugar, salt, chemicals and industrial oils like canola and corn oil is highly pro inflammatory. Inflammation in turn causes stress, pain and disease, which in turn drain the body of important nutrients. When you are stressed, you need double the amount of vitamins necessary in a calm state. Even eating well might not cover that amount so imagine what a junk food diet does to your health.

The modern diet is also lacking in vitamins like the B vitamins, vitamin C and vitamin D, and minerals like magnesium, potassium and chromium. All of this can be related to adrenal fatigue, chronic fatigue, stress, general pain and stiffness, irritability and of course, sleep problems.

Things like sugar, alcohol, caffeine, phosphates (in sodas) and certain medications (birth control pills, diuretics, insulin, and antibiotics) cause the loss of vitamins and minerals, especially magnesium. Magnesium is absolutely essential for life and is known as the relaxation mineral. Unsurprisingly, it is helpful for insomnia, restless leg syndrome, sore muscles, arthritis and aches and pains.

Getting enough magnesium in your diet is fairly difficult because our soil has become depleted in this important mineral. Magnesium oil (magnesium chloride) or Epsom salts (magnesium sulfate) are both good ways to get magnesium through the skin.

Bananas are a good source and they also have potassium. Potassium too helps with nerve relaxation and there seems to be an intriguing link between the mineral and delta sleep—the deep relaxing and restorative sleep.

> *Take an Epsom salts bath to relieve pain, relax sore and tired muscles and ensure a good night's sleep. Dissolve one cup of Epsom salts, aka magnesium sulfate, in a hot bath to help draw impurities out of your body and allow you to absorb magnesium transdermally. Soak for 20 minutes, drink a glass of water and go to bed.*

The best diet overall for sleep would be an anti-inflammatory diet. This would be high in vegetables, especially the green leafy kind, and good fats like avocados, nuts, butter, fatty fish, chia and flax seeds, olives and extra virgin olive oil and devoid of simple sugars, white flour products and anything artificial and or processed. Cocoa, berries, and the herbs and spices such as cinnamon, ginger, turmeric, garlic, oregano and basil are all loaded with antioxidants and anti-inflammatory agents.

Stress

Stress can stop you from getting a good night's sleep but poor sleep can contribute to stress and so you have the classic vicious circle which continues to feed itself. Unfortunately, high stress also makes you a bit stupid because it cuts you off from the rational part of your brain.

Physical stress comes from eating an inflammatory diet, lack of exercise and lack of sleep. Mental and psychological stress comes from the thoughts we think and our left brained society with its focus on getting, spending, doing and accumulating, which of course encourages us to work harder and sleep less. We need to turn the tables and do exactly the opposite.

Compartmentalized

You might have noticed a trend here. Chronic light, chronic sitting, chronic thinking, chronic diseases–if we are not careful, our lives can slip into the grey middling zone where there's no dark to counteract the light, no movement to counteract the sitting, no meditation and quiet time to counteract the thinking and no health to counteract disease.

There's no yang because there's no yin. Relying on sleep as a catchall off switch to magically restore us physically, mentally and emotionally is just wishful thinking. Sleep can restore us but only when we accord sleep the respect it deserves instead of treating it as a standalone activity disconnected from the rest of our lives.

Instead of compartmentalizing everything we do from sleep to diet, health, relationships, work and exercise, we need to see how everything fits into and influences everything else. If you don't expend some energy in vigorous exercise, sleep won't be as restful as it could be. If you don't take time to unwind your brain, by the time you lie down, those whizzing thoughts could prevent sleep. If you eat all day and don't give your digestion a rest, it will interfere with sleep.

Then the lack of good sleep will feed into other parts of your life, making you less productive at work, less effective in relationships, more anxious and less energetic. This leads to eating more carbs, putting on more weight, feeling less inclined to exercise and ultimately more stressed, which makes sleep harder to come by and so on and so on.

> *make it dark, cool and quiet*

Tips for good sleep hygiene:

We can sum up good sleep hygiene in three words: dark, cool and quiet.

➢ Make your bedroom a device-free room to avoid sleep procrastination–you know how it goes, just one more cat video on YouTube and then you'll go to bed. Alternatively, keep the charger in another room as this will prevent you from surfing mindlessly for hours because you are more likely to just go to bed than fetch the charger when the battery runs down.

➢ Do not use your bed for anything other than sleeping and intimacy. If you work, watch TV or play computer games in bed, there's just way too much activity associated with it. You want your bed to represent a peaceful haven of sleep only.

➢ For the same reason, if you are not asleep after 15 minutes, get up, do something calming for 20-30 minutes and go back to bed.

➢ Make sure the temperature is set at about 69° or lower.

➤ If there is a lot of outside light from street lights etc., use blackout curtains in your bedroom.

➤ If you get up in the middle of the night to use the bathroom, try not to switch the light on. If you have to have a light, make sure it's not a bright one.

➤ Install software on your devices that change the color the screens emit by muting or changing the blue light.

➤ Wear blue blocking glasses at night to protect your eyes from high energy short wavelength light.

➤ Instead of looking at a computer or TV screen at night, listen to audiobooks or music.

➤ Do something relaxing to wind down before bed—reading, journaling, knitting, prayer, music, etc.

➤ Two hours before bed, turn off all your devices and start transitioning from daytime activities to night time ones.

➤ Don't eat anything or do strenuous exercise less than three hours before bedtime.

➤ Make sure you get exposure to bright, natural light during the day light.

➤ Replace LED/fluorescent lights with incandescent bulbs or dim red lights, especially in your bedroom.

- ➤ Alternatively, use a Himalayan salt lamp–it is kinder on the eyes and it will also neutralize positive ions in the air.

- ➤ Establish a sleep routine and try to stick to it every day, including weekends.

- ➤ Waking up at the same time every day helps you sleep more efficiently because your body knows to prepare for waking at the same time every day.

- ➤ Empty your brain on to paper before you go to bed so you don't worry about forgetting something important.

- ➤ If you find yourself lying there in bed ruminating and worrying about what you have to do the next day, get up and write it down and go back to bed.

- ➤ Learn meditation or mindfulness. Both are simple to learn but hard to practice but will help calm the monkey mind and therefore improve sleep.

- ➤ Invest in a good sleep system.

You probably already know instinctively what would help you to sleep better but chances are you simply don't have the motivation to do it. Instead of trying to use willpower to white knuckle your way to better sleep and better health, you would do well to set up better habits. This removes your thinking brain from the equation and helps you move in the direction you want to go.

Section 3:

The Sleep System

What is a Sleep System?

If you have never heard of the term "Sleep System", let us explain. A sleep system is a combination of comfort and support products that will help you fall asleep faster, stay asleep longer and wake up more refreshed. Before you assume that *sleep system* is just the fancy way of saying bed, like *home engineer* is the fancy way of saying *housewife*, let us remind you that a third of your life is spent horizontally.

In the same way as the sacred work of women in the home cannot be fairly summed up by saying 'just a housewife', building a sleep system is very different than simply looking for a "good" mattress. Building your life around sleep requires investing in your own custom sleep system. This system requires professional fitting by a bedding expert or "sleep engineer" as we like to call ourselves.

Goldilocks in the bedroom

We live in an increasingly technical age and sometimes that is not such a good thing but in sleep merchandise it means there is so much choice, innovation and progress. Unfortunately, it also means overwhelm for the average consumer. When it comes to choosing how to configure your sleeping requirements, find an expert you can trust to help you find something that is not too hard and not too soft but just right.

> *"Life is too short to sleep on low thread-count sheets." ~Leah Stussy*

Sleep System in a nutshell:

A good quality Sleep System addresses four main areas:

1. Support

2. Pressure relief

3. Temperature regulation

4. Motion transfer:

and consists of:

1. Queen size Sleep Pillow,

2.   High Quality Mattress

3.   Adjustable, aka Lifestyle, Base

4.   Temperature Regulated Sheets

5.   Breathable Mattress Protector

Support

One of the most important aspects of your sleep system is support, which should not be confused with firmness. Good support allows different parts of your body to sink into the surface of the mattress whilst other parts are maintained in a comfortable position. All of this is governed by how your body interacts with the different layers that make up a mattress, your unique sleeping preferences and sleeping style.

Make sure your sleep consultant understands things like the mechanisms of progressive resistance so they can help you choose the perfect recipe to suit your individual requirements.

As a quarter of the sleep surface consists of your pillow, finding one that is right for you is crucial. Your head is largely responsible for telling your body if it is comfortable but it's difficult to see where the problem is when you are uncomfortable because you can't see yourself. Here a knowledgeable sleep consultant is invaluable because they have the experience to combine the visual aspect with the right solution. They can show you where your spine is badly aligned or where you have gaps that should not be there, like under the lumbar spine.

Pressure relief

This refers to how a specific material responds to the shape of the body. If it offers good pressure relief, it is able to absorb and redistribute the weight from certain areas so that there is no undue pressure on them and you get a more comfortable sleep experience. This also allows you to sleep more efficiently as you get to sleep through all five cycles.

Generally, when people think about pressure relief, they think memory foam. Whilst memory foam can be a very comfortable solution, either in isolation or in combination with other pressure relieving materials, it has a tremendous amount of health and sleep benefits because memory foam allows you to comfortably stay in the same position throughout the sleep cycles and get deep restorative sleep. Make sure to consult an expert who can walk you through the pros and cons of different materials in this regard.

Temperature regulation

The right materials regulate temperature so that you don't get too hot or too cold, both of which would disrupt sleep. Careful consideration should be given to the sheets and pillow cases that come into direct contact with your skin, as well as the textiles used in the layers immediately under them. Different materials have differing abilities to wick away moisture and heat and so will affect sleep positively or negatively. You need someone who can cut through all the jargon and give you the best advice. The styling is as important as the fabric because, for instance, a badly fitting sheet can affect the way your mattress behaves.

Motion transfer

There's probably nothing more annoying than being disturbed in sleep every time your partner moves, especially if you are a light sleeper. This can be a real problem for those who cohabit with a restless sleeper who fidgets or flings themselves around a lot. There are plenty of choices of beds that help isolate movements so they don't spread around and disturb you and the other sleeper but finding the right fit is a bit of a balancing act where good guidance is a must.

Section 4:

Putting the Sleep Myths to Bed

Myth No. 1: We all need 8 hours sleep a night

> *"The amount of sleep required by the average person is five minutes more."* ~ Wilson Mizener

This advice, which has become more of an edict of late, is on a par with telling everyone they should drink eight glasses of water or consume 2,000 calories a day. Yes, we should all sleep, drink and eat enough but how much is enough? Enough for one person might be too much for another and nowhere near enough for yet another. Margaret Thatcher is famously known for sleeping only four hours a night, successful fashion designer Tom Ford needs only three and apparently Tesla survived on a paltry two.

There are many more examples of people who function very well on much less sleep than the official guidelines and there seems to be a scientific reason for this. A very small percentage of the population have what has been dubbed the "Thatcher gene". Less than 1% of us have the short sleep variation of the BHLHE41 gene.

In a press release announcing the discovery of the mutant gene, American Academy of Sleep Medicine President, Dr. Timothy Morgenthaler, is quoted as saying, "This study emphasizes that our need for sleep is a biological requirement, not a personal preference". [16]

At the other end of the spectrum are the long sleepers who make up about 6% of the population. Their biological requirement is way more than the allotted eight hours. For instance, Einstein liked to sleep for ten hours or more every night, supplemented with daytime naps. Model Heidi Klum insists on getting ten hours and singer Mariah Carey says she needs 15.

In light of the fact that humans are such an amazingly diverse bunch, the eight-hour rule seems a bit arbitrary. So how much sleep do you need? It depends, and only you can answer that question. The simple answer is the amount you need is the amount you need. The thing is, even if your base line is eight hours a night, if you are sick, stressed, overworked or lacking in essential nutrients, you may need more. Once you have caught up, you can

---

[16] http://www.aasmnet.org/articles.aspx?id=4899

go back to sleeping eight hours again.

If you wake up without an alarm clock feeling bright eyed and bushy tailed after six hours of sleep, you have had enough sleep. If you sleep for ten hours and feel like death when you wake up, either you are not sleeping enough or the quality of your sleep is bad. Alternatively, there might be something else going on in your life that needs attention. Either way, trying to fit into some cookie cutter notion of sleep is not going to help you.

This puts a different spin on sleep and puts it into the context of your life as a whole instead of something separate that you evaluate in terms of a number. If you want to find out the optimal amount of sleep for you, the best way to go about it is to wake up at the same time every single day. At night, your body will let you know when you need to go to bed because you will feel tired. When the routine becomes an established part of your life, your body will automatically adjust when you need to go to sleep so that you can wake up at the time it has come to expect in the morning.

As long as you don't ignore the tiredness at night by pushing beyond it, you should be able to find a sleep rhythm that suits you. Of course, this approach entails being able to listen to your body, something not encouraged in the age of "speak to your doctor" about everything from what vitamins to take to what exercise you should do. Doctors don't study health, vitamins, nutrition or exercise and they get little to no training in sleep. Doctors study disease and their solutions most often come in the form of drugs.

> *"We've all been told you ought to sleep 8 hr., but there was never any evidence." ~ Dr. Daniel Kripke*

In 2002, the National Sleep Foundation was recommending that adults get eight hours of sleep. By 2015, this had been extended to 7-9 hours. This all sounds very reasonable until you look at the results of the largest sleep study in history, incorporating 1.1 million men and women between the ages of 30 and 102.

This was the first study large enough to differentiate between seven and eight hours and the conclusion was: "The best survival was found among those who slept 7 hours per night. Participants who reported sleeping 8 hours or more experienced significantly increased mortality hazard, as did those who slept 6 hours or less. The increased risk exceeded 15% for those reporting more than 8.5 hours sleep or less than 3.5 or 4.5 hours." [17] These results were later replicated in Asia and Europe.

Lead author of the study, Professor Daniel F. Kripke, later said in an interview with Time, "There is just as much risk associated with sleeping too long as with sleeping too short. The big surprise is that long sleep seems to start at

---

[17] http://www.ncbi.nlm.nih.gov/pubmed/11825133

8 hr. Sleeping 8.5 hr. might really be a little worse than sleeping 5 hr." [18]

He goes on to say "One of the reasons I like to publicize these facts is that I think we can prevent a lot of insomnia and distress just by telling people that short sleep is O.K. We've all been told you ought to sleep 8 hr., but there was never any evidence." He says that in an effort to sleep the requisite eight to nine hours, people end up spending too long in bed "with the result that they have trouble falling asleep and wake up a lot during the night. Oddly enough, a lot of the problem [of insomnia] is lying in bed awake, worrying about it. There have been many controlled studies in the U.S., Great Britain and other parts of Europe that show that an insomnia treatment that involves getting out of bed when you're not sleepy and restricting your time in bed actually helps people to sleep more."

In effect, when people stop trying to fit a square peg into a round hole, they stop fearing their bed. The lack of sleep becomes a non-issue because they know when they do go to bed, they will actually sleep instead of just lying there tossing and turning. "So spending less time in bed actually makes sleep better. It is in fact a more powerful and effective long-term treatment for insomnia than sleeping pills." This brings us to the subject of sleep medication and how the eight hour myth came about.

---

[18] http://content.time.com/time/health/article/0,8599,1812420,00.html

Myth No. 2: Sleeping pills help you sleep

They really don't but before we get into that, we need to understand why people believe they do. Again, we have Dr. Kripke to thank for shedding some light on the issue. In an article published in the Huffington post in 2016, he muses, "You might wonder why for over 20 years the NSF has been advising adults to sleep 8 hours, when those who sleep 6-7 hours live longer and suffer less cardiovascular deaths. Could it be that crying wolf about long sleep might not sell sleeping pills as well as fear of short sleep?"

It turns out that the major sponsors for the launch of The National Sleep Foundation (NSF) were the manufacturers of sleeping pills and these manufacturers continue to fund the non-profit organization. In 1993, the makers of Ambien launched a $60 million advertising and marketing campaign which dovetailed very nicely with the NSF's campaign "to raise insomnia to its deserved level of a national public health crisis." This was accompanied by the ubiquitous "speak to your doctor" mantra and Ambien turned into a blockbuster drug. A subsequent campaign by the NSF resulted in a huge uptick of hypnotics prescribed for children.

When pharmaceutical companies embark on a marketing crusade for a new drug, they don't just try to educate the public. They spend a considerable amount of time, effort and money on educating those who will be prescribing the drugs, namely the doctors. This could explain why, in the 15 years between 1993 and 2007, prescriptions for nonbenzodiazepine sedative hypnotics (e.g. Ambien/zolpidem) expanded "21 times more rapidly than did sleeplessness complaints and 5 times more rapidly than did insomnia diagnoses, suggesting that life problems are being treated with medical solutions". This is from a study examining the trends in sleeplessness complaints, diagnoses, and prescriptions of sedative hypnotics, *The Medicalization of Sleeplessness: A Public Health Concern* [19] . The authors noted "It is unclear, however, if the United States is facing a true insomnia epidemic or a surplus of diagnoses and drug prescriptions."

Kripke, who has been in the business of sleep for over 40 years, says, "If you worry about short sleep, do NOT take sleeping pills. Worldwide, there have now been 40 epidemiologic studies of the mortality risks associated with taking sleeping pills, of which 39 showed that people taking sleeping pills died sooner." [20]

In his book *The Dark Side of Sleeping Pills,* he talks about a study comparing 10,000 plus patients who took sleeping pills with more than 20,000 matched patients who did not. In the 2.5 year follow-up, those taking the pills died 4.6 times more often than those not taking them and those taking higher doses died 5.3 times more. "Even those patients who took fewer than 18 pills per year had

---

[19] https://www.ncbi.nlm.nih.gov/pmc/articles/PMC3134490/

[20] http://www.huffingtonpost.com/daniel-f-kripke-md/is-short-sleep-a-big-bad-_b_9731824.html

very significantly elevated mortality, 3.6 times that of patients who took no hypnotics." [20]

Sleep medications increase the risk of depression, infection, sleep apnea, dependence, daytime sleepiness, and death from overdose, especially in combination with opiates. Among their side effects are sleep walking, sleep driving and sleep eating. But do they increase sleep? Yes, by an average of 11 minutes. They also help you get to sleep about 13 minutes sooner. Drugs like Ambien (and Valium and Xanax) have sedative effects which appear to help you sleep but actually prevent deep sleep.

Despite the fact that sleep medications don't really work that well, most people who take them are convinced otherwise. Perhaps this is because most sleeping pills reduce anxiety. If you're not getting great sleep but you're not particularly worried about it, all's good. And then there's anterograde amnesia, the forgetfulness induced by most sleeping pills. You might have horrible fragmented sleep but the medication prevents you from forming memories so when you wake up in the morning, you don't even remember how badly you slept.

The other huge problem with sleep medication is that it catastrophizes something that should be a natural biological imperative and reduces it to a pharmaceutical problem. Once you take a pill to help you sleep, you stop looking at why you couldn't sleep in the first place.

---

[21] http://www.darksideofsleepingpills.com/index.html

Sleeping pills are also addictive and sometimes the withdrawal symptoms are far worse than the insomnia which might have prompted you to take them in the first place.

> *"The magic pill for sleep has not been invented yet." ~ Dr. Manisha Witmans (sleep medicine specialist at the University of Alberta's Evidence-Based Practice Center)* [22]

Myth No. 3: There's an epidemic of sleep deprivation and we are getting less sleep than we used to

This one is tricky because there is no denying that there is something amiss with our relationship to sleep. Some experts say we are sleeping an hour or so less than we did a couple of centuries ago. Others disagree, pointing out that as we no longer have to deal with sleep disruptors like bed bugs, sleeping on primitive beds or no beds, sleeping with the whole family and maybe a cow or two, freezing temperatures and the threat of wild animals or fires.

We have no way of going back into the distant past to study the sleep habits of our ancestors but researchers

---

[22] http://www.nytimes.com/2007/10/23/health/23drug.html?pagewanted=all&_r=0

came up with an ingenious solution and tracked the sleep of three pre-industrial societies instead. They studied hunter-gatherers who live traditionally and without electricity or the trappings of civilization and published their results in 2015 in a paper entitled *Natural sleep and its seasonal variations in three pre-industrial societies.* [23]

The researchers used wrist devices to record sleep time, temperature and light exposure in groups from the Tsimane in Bolivia, the Hadza in Tanzania and the San people in Namibia and found "all three show similar sleep organization, suggesting that they express core human sleep patterns, likely characteristic of pre-modern era Homo sapiens."

A number of surprises was in store for the researchers. One, the average sleep time for the tribespeople was between 5.7 to 7.1 hours a night, a full hour or two less than we have been led to believe is optimal. Yet all three groups were found to be physically fitter and healthier than people in industrialized societies with no obesity or blood pressure issues. They all fell asleep easily and insomnia was almost unheard of. Two of the groups did not even have the equivalent word for it in their languages.

Two, none of them hit the sack the moment the sun went down but lingered around the fire talking, dancing and

---

[23] https://www.ncbi.nlm.nih.gov/pmc/articles/PMC4720388/

eating until more than three hours later. They generally were up before dawn the next morning, except for the San who rose an hour after dawn in the summer. Temperature, rather than light seemed to regulate the amount and timing of sleep. All groups, however, received a large amount of natural light exposure in the mornings and slept in darkness.

So are we getting less sleep than our ancestors did? Probably not but the real question is are we getting enough quality sleep for the lifestyles we lead? There's no comparison between the frenetic pace of our lives and the calm traditional pace of hunter-gatherers who live in tune with the rhythms of the seasons.

Professor Jim Horne, former director of Loughborough University's Sleep Research Centre, also talks about "core sleep". This is the first five hours of normal sleep, which seems to be "the sleep most beneficial to the slumbering cortex." Over the next hour, this sleep gradually disappears and so by the end of six hours has generally been replaced by what he calls "optional" or "elastic" sleep, which is where we stay until we wake up. The optional sleep isn't really optional but more flexible than core sleep. [24]

This brings us to the next myth about sleep being a rigid construct.

---

[24] http://www.lboro.ac.uk/departments/ssehs/research/behavioural-medicine/sleep-research-centre/keyinterests/name-45025-en.html

Myth no. 4: There's only one way to sleep

You would think that sleep is just a case of putting your head on the pillow, sleeping for x amount of hours and then getting up in the morning, having slept. It turns out that the way we treat sleep in the 21st century is quite different to the way it was treated hundreds of years ago. Moreover, there's more than one way to skin a sleeping cat and there are different ways of manipulating the time you have to get the sleep you need.

We are accustomed to monophasic sleep where we expect to get all our sleep in one big chunk. The idea of biphasic sleep (sleep in two stages) or polyphasic sleep (sleep in multiple stages) is so foreign to most of us that we'd consider either of them as unnatural or just plain weird. Looking at what we would consider atypical sleeping methods challenges our concept of normal and acceptable sleep.

The Da Vinci Sleep Schedule: Also known as the "Uberman" sleep, this was allegedly perfected by the Italian polymath Leonardo da Vinci. Da Vinci slept at least 20 minutes to no more than two hours roughly every four hours to net around 21 hours of awake time out of every 24. The polyphasic sleep pattern allowed him to sustain an incredible output of work without being inactive for any appreciable length of time.

Obviously this is quite extreme and not for the faint hearted but there are some people who have managed to get it right in the 21st century. Apparently boredom and loneliness drive them back to 'normal' sleep. One of the problems they encounter is that unless they stick to a very rigid pattern and miss a sleep, it throws out the whole game and they feel awful. As a controversial and anti-social sleep method, it is not recommended but just thinking about it stretches our idea of what is possible. After all, many animals sleep polyphasically, just as we all did as babies.

Two Sleeps: Once upon a time, about 200-300 years ago, getting up in the middle of the night and entertaining visitors, praying, having sex or doing a bit of meditation was perfectly normal behavior because that's what everyone else was doing. Then, it was known as wakefulness but if you do that now, you're an insomniac. Biphasic sleep was not in evidence in the hunter-gatherer societies mentioned earlier and it is thought that the pattern developed in colder climates far from the equator—someone had to get up to stoke the fire at night. Taking a regular siesta in the afternoon can also be considered a form of biphasic sleep.

Literature from a few hundred years ago reflected 'first sleep' at about 9pm and 'second sleep' commencing after a break of an hour or so around midnight and lasting until daybreak. With the advent of street lights and nightlife, this gradually fell out of fashion and vanished from our consciousness. Our sleep became the compressed monophasic pattern we have all come to regard as the one and only correct way to sleep today.

The Nap: Not so long ago, you did not want to be caught napping but then the practice was rescued by reinvention and became the power nap. John F. Kennedy napped for an hour or two in the middle of every day. No one interrupted his naptime. Churchill napped, Napoleon napped and Darwin napped. Churchill even had a bed in the Houses of Parliament and relied on his naps as essential elements to power nap his way through a challenging leadership.

One study from California studied the relationship between naps and workers for 25 years. They found 92.5% of workers increased productivity, creativity and problem-solving skills after a short afternoon nap.

Section 5:

The Spiritual Aspect of Sleep

> *"The dream is the small hidden door in the deepest and most intimate sanctum of the soul, which opens to that primeval cosmic night that was soul long before there was conscious ego and will be soul far beyond what a conscious ego could ever reach."* ~ *Carl Jung*

This section is a circling back to the beginning of the book where we talked about sleep belonging to the imaginative, emotional domain and how it has been demoted in a sense by the logical, analytical one. As a mere part of sleep, dreams have been demoted lower still.

To the rational mind, dreams are nothing special and just the result of random neural activity conjuring up vibrant images of things happening only on the screen of the imagination. What if this was completely wrong in the same way that scientists labelled most of our DNA (roughly 97% of it) as "junk" simply because they hadn't figured out what it was for?

If you were to unravel the tightly coiled DNA of a single human cell, it would stretch to about ten feet but researchers discovered only a tiny percentage of it encoded genes and the vast stretches in between and around the genes appeared redundant. Surely such large chunks of genetic material would not be faithfully replicated and conserved over millions of years if it served no purpose. Now it seems that those stretches influence how genes behave because they are filled with teeny-weeny genetic switches.

This information emerged from the torrent of data generated between 2007-2012 by more than 400 geneticists involved in the international ENCODE (ENCyclopedia Of DNA Elements) project. At the time, Ewan Birney, who was responsible for coordinating the massive amount of data, said, "I get this strong feeling that previously I was ignorant of my own ignorance, and now I understand my ignorance. It's slightly depressing as you realize how ignorant you are...Ten years ago we didn't know what we didn't know." [25]

By the same token, we don't know what we don't know about dreams and can therefore speculate that the plus minus 200,000 dreams the average person could

---

[25] https://www.scientificamerican.com/article/hidden-treasures-in-junk-dna/

experience by the time they hit age 60 are valuable in some profound way. Analyzing the 15 trillion bytes of raw data to make some sense of the "dark matter" of human DNA equated to over three centuries of computer time and they still can't tell us a whole lot about it. Dreams are far more ephemeral and even more difficult to pin down than DNA so what chance is there that we can begin to understand them from the current paradigm of "what can't be measured, can't exist"?

If we want to understand dreams from an entirely different paradigm, we have to delve into the bizarre world of quantum mechanics (QM), which is as mind-bendingly peculiar as dreams themselves. Einstein found it so disconcerting that he preferred not to think about it and referred to it as "spooky actions at a distance."

> *"Anyone not shocked by quantum mechanics has not yet understood it." ~ Niels Bohr*

Quantum mechanics describes what happens at the level of the atomic and subatomic where objects can be particles and waves and exist in many different places at the same time. Within this domain is the MWI (Many Worlds Interpretation), a hypothesis which states that different versions of you occupy an infinite number of worlds that are constantly splitting off with each miniscule divergence. Therefore, we inhabit a multiverse and we are not so much individuals but multiplicities with an exponential number of possible versions of ourselves.

Probably the most disturbing thing about QM, which paradoxically helps ease the weirdness of the MWI, is the revelation that atoms are mostly voids. They are full of nothing, they are empty except for an itty bitty nucleus, which is where almost all (99.7%) of their mass is concentrated, surrounded by orbiting electrons, aka the electron cloud. But the nucleus is impossibly small compared to the atom. To put it in perspective, if the nucleus was the same size as a football stadium, the atom would be the size of planet Earth. If the electron cloud was the size of a football stadium, the nucleus would be akin to a mosquito in the middle of the stadium.

We are made up of atoms, the basic building blocks of matter, just like a table, a rock and every other thing on the planet is, which means we are mostly hot air, or at least mostly empty space. The substance or solidity we suppose exists, does not–it merely appears to exist because that's what our brains telling us. When we see, hear, touch, taste or smell anything, we are not actually seeing, hearing, touching, tasting or smelling anything but rather experiencing our brains interpretation of the sense data. Here's another huge paradox, which, by the by, is the main teaching tool of spiritual inquiry and religion.

If we are mostly empty, what are we then? Ancient wisdom tells us, and cutting edge science like superstring theory has confirmed it, we are vibration and energy. Vibration links us to everything else, including the table and the rock–vibrations are at the core of all existence. Right now, most of us don't know that we can pick up on vibration and energy because we were never taught to do it.

> *"To 'see both sides' of a problem is the surest way to prevent its complete solution. Because there are always more than two sides." ~ Idries Shah*

There is nothing straightforward about quantum mechanics. In *From Eternity to Here*, Sean Carroll writes, "We're still not sure what is the best way to think and talk about quantum mechanics.

This interpretational anxiety stems from the single basic difference between quantum mechanics and classical mechanics, which is both simple and world-shattering in its implications:

According to quantum mechanics, what we can observe about the world is only a tiny subset of what actually exists." [26]

The incontrovertible conclusion is that we are living in a self-aware universe where time and space do not exist.

---

[26] http://www.preposterousuniverse.com/eternitytohere/quantum/

Nothing is separate from anything else and whatever happened in the past or will happen in the future is happening now at this very moment. It's like Groundhog Day on a humungous scale and it makes us all immortal because we existed before we were born and continue to exist after we die.

According to Chad Orzel, Associate Professor in the Department of Physics and Astronomy at Union College, the MWI is merely a metaphor to get around the 'measurement problem' which would otherwise interfere with the validity of quantum mechanics. He says, "Quantum physics deals in probabilities, not certainty, and the mathematical wavefunctions we calculate within the theory will contain pieces describing multiple possible outcomes right up until the moment of measurement. And yet, we experience only a single reality, with any given measurement having one and only one outcome." [27]

But then there's this from the Book of Mormon, in Moses 1:33, where God says "And worlds without number have I created;" and this from the Quran 1:2, "All praise is due to God alone, the Sustainer of all the worlds". Hebrew Scripture references "an infinite number of worlds, of physical, spiritual and inter-dimensional nature."

Both Buddhism and Hinduism make mention of infinite

---

[27] https://www.forbes.com/sites/chadorzel/2016/01/05/what-the-many-worlds-interpreta-tion-of-quantum-physics-really-means/#43d289f41102

worlds and innumerable universes. For instance, in the Hindu *Bhagavata Purana* we find: "Every universe is covered by seven layers — earth, water, fire, air, sky, the total energy and false ego — each ten times greater than the previous one. There are innumerable universes besides this one, and although they are unlimitedly large, they move about like atoms in You. Therefore You are called unlimited." [28]

Thus, as strange as quantum logic sounds, it is nothing new. This brings us back, seemingly by way of Japan, to dreams. Dreams are a mystery within the bigger mystery of sleep but only because we have accepted wakefulness as the default. If our bodies are mostly empty space that we only perceive as flesh and blood, what does being awake actually mean other than a simulation looping endlessly in order for us to experience, grow and learn? If this is so, time and space become irrelevant and the notion of a multiverse makes perfect sense.

> *Jesus said, "The kingdom of God does not come with observation; nor will they say, 'See here!' or 'See there!' For indeed, the kingdom of God is within you" (Luke 17:20-21)*

To be awake is to be aware. Aware of what? Are you aware of the nature of your own mind? Generally, when

---

[28] http://www.jewishmag.com/8mag/worlds/worlds1.htm

we talk about awareness, it is with relation to the outside world. When you are asleep, that awareness fades but you can still be aware of (awake to) another world–the vaster world within.

> *"Our truest life is when we are in dreams awake." ~ Thoreau*

So, we have established what we think of as real is just an interpretation, being 'awake' in this false reality is the illusion, and the dream world is an alternate but possibly more valid reality. If we accept all this, we can appreciate what mystical thinking and indigenous people have been saying all along. People like the Hopi Indians and Australian Aboriginies have always maintained that so-called reality is the illusion/dream and one day we will wake up or become enlightened.

In the meantime, however, humanity is for the most part asleep and in answer to the question of what he thought was man's fundamental mistake, Sufi Idries Shah said, "To think that he is alive, when he has merely fallen asleep in life's waiting room."

According to the doctrines of Sufism, the mystical Islamic search for divine truth, there are seven levels of the self, ascending from the purely egotistical to the purely spiritual. Robert Frager, Founder of the Institute for Transpersonal Psychology and writer on Sufism, says in an article called *Transforming the Self*, "The lowest level of the self, the ego or lower personality, is made up of impulses, or drives, to satisfy desires. These drives dominate reason or judgment and are defined as the forces in one's nature that must be brought under control. The self is a product of the self-centered consciousness - the ego, the "I." The self must be transformed - this is the ideal. The self is like a wild horse; it is powerful and virtually uncontrollable. As the self becomes trained, or transformed, it becomes capable of serving the individual." [29]

> "You have not forgotten to remember;
> You have remembered to forget.
> But people can forget to forget. That is just
> as important as remembering to remember–
> and generally more practical." ~ Idries Shah,
> Reflections

One of the defining attributes of dreaming in REM sleep is the dissolving of the ego.

According to the ancient wisdom of the Hindus, our waking life is just a projection of the movies we choose to play upon the screen of consciousness. To ascend to higher levels of consciousness, we first have to recognize that projection by awakening or, put another way, by increasing our awareness of our place in the cosmos.

---

[29] http://www.katinkahesselink.net/sufi/sufi.htm

Eckhart Tolle says, "You are not IN the universe, you ARE the universe, an intrinsic part of it. Ultimately you are not a person, but a focal point where the universe is becoming conscious of itself."

New Age meets Ancient Egypt in Dreams

> *"I dream, therefore I exist." ~ August Strindberg, A Madman's Defense*

Dream travel, trained dreamers, lucid dreaming, remote viewing, dream guides, dream school, sleep temple, dream diary and the Magic Library all seem to be phrases that would fit right in with some New Agey symposium on astral traveling. They are in fact from an article about ancient Egyptians called *Dreaming like an Egyptian*, written by Robert Moss, who describes himself as "a dream teacher, on a path for which there has been no career track in our culture." [30]

Moss is a former lecturer in ancient history at the Australian National University and he travels all over the world teaching Active Dreaming, an original synthesis of dreamwork and shamanism. He writes, "Through conscious dream travel, ancient Egypt's 'frequent flyers' explored the roads of the afterlife and the

---

[30] http://www.beliefnet.com/columnists/dreamgates/2010/10/dreaming-like-an-egyptian.html#aHKQJMaPaL5ZPX0g.99A

multidimensional universe. It was understood that true initiation and transformation takes place in a deeper reality accessible through the dream journey beyond the body." [31]

The ancient Egyptian word for sleep (qed) was represented by the symbol of a bed. Dream (rswt or resut) was represented by the symbol of an open eye and rswt literally means to come awake. In hieroglyphics, dream is written by combining the symbol of an open eye with the symbol of a bed, clearly illustrating that Egyptians thought dreaming was to awaken in sleep. This could also have been denoting the state of consciousness that we now call lucid dreaming.

The Magic Library was the Egyptian's way of referring to the land of nod and dreaming was so important to the Egyptians that they had priests dedicated to dreaming called the Learned Ones of the Magic Library. Ancient Egypt had many sleep temples, better understood by us as hospitals, where sleep therapy and sleep medicine was performed.

In a paper by Dr. Tarek Asaad, *Sleep in Ancient Egypt* [32], he says:

---

[31] http://www.beliefnet.com/columnists/dreamgates/2010/10/dreaming-like-an-egyptian.html#aHKQJMaPaL5ZPX0g.99

[32] link.springer.com/chapter/10.1007%2F978-1-4939-2089-1_2

"Ancient Egyptians believed each person has five bodies:

1. ka=creative or divine power or the living physical body

2. ba=soul, able to travel beyond the physical body

3. akh or Shat=body of the deceased in the afterlife (the corpse body) which means the union of the ka and ba

4. the name=living part of the person

5. the shadow=another living part of the person

This description of multidimensional levels of the self has something to do with sleep, as the ancient Egyptians believed in the ability of the ba (soul) to travel beyond the physical body during sleep. The ba was represented in hieroglyphics as a human-headed bird floating above the sleeping body. In that sense, sleep was viewed to be similar, in some aspect, to death, in which the person is in a different state or a different world. Being strong believers in the afterlife, sleep was considered as a way or outlet to that mysterious world and a means through which a person can communicate with the dead as well as his gods. For this reason, it is not surprising to find some rituals related to sleep to resemble what is adopted in preparation for death."

Hypnosis and Dream Cures

We like to think of hypnosis as some modern invention but it has its roots in many ancient civilizations from the Druids to the Greeks, Egyptians, Chinese and Tibetans. The history of hypnosis is entwined with the history of sleep and hypnosis trance states and deep sleep were all intertwined in religious, spiritual and medicinal practices, perhaps through every culture since the beginning of time. The first recorded use of hypnosis comes from over 5,000 years ago in the Egypt's Old Kingdom.

Imhotep, chancellor and high priest of the sun god Ra, initiated the tradition of "temple sleep" where the sick would visit the temple to find a cure from the gods in sleep. After hours of ritual chanting and ingestion of herbs, they would lie down in darkened chambers to await dreams, which were then analyzed for the cure.

Shamanism and Schizophrenia

The state of dreaming has been described as one in which you can go safely insane. It's like having a psychotic episode full of hallucinations where you are delusional, disorientated, paralyzed and emotionally unstable with a bit of amnesia thrown in for good measure. When you dream, you generally do not know that you are dreaming, regardless of how bizarre or random the dream is because activity in the prefrontal cortex declines. This part of the brain is command central for logic, planning and regulating social behavior.

In other words, it is being out of touch with 'reality' or pretty close to what would be described as being schizophrenic. In an interview with Melvyn Bragg discussing the interpretation of dreams, Mark Solms, Professor of Neuropsychology at the University of Cape Town, says, "The neurochemistry and neuroanatomy of dreams has striking overlaps with what we know of the neurochemistry and neuroanatomy of schizophrenia." [33] In fact, it has been hypothesized that *schizophrenia is waking reality processed through the dreaming brain.* [34]

In our society, schizophrenia is the cancer of mental health and nobody wants that kind of diagnosis. In other cultures however, people don't seem to have the same kind of negative and phobic response to the auditory and visual hallucinations which are common features of schizophrenia. In one study, researchers discovered that while "many of the African and Indian subjects registered predominantly positive experiences with their voices, not one American did. Rather, the U.S. subjects were more likely to report experiences as violent and hateful—and evidence of a sick condition." [35]

In a lecture given in 1994, Terence McKenna said, "A shaman is someone who swims in the same ocean as the schizophrenic, but the shaman has thousands and

[33] http://www.bbc.co.uk/programmes/p004y23x

[34] http://www.bmj.com/rapid-response/2011/11/01/schizophrenia-waking-reality-processed-through-dreaming-brain

[35] https://www.theatlantic.com/health/archive/2014/07/when-hearing-voices-is-a-good-thing/374863/

thousands of years of sanctioned technique and tradition to draw upon. In a traditional society, if you exhibited 'schizophrenic' tendencies, you are immediately drawn out of the pack and put under the care and tutelage of master shamans. You are told: 'You are special. Your abilities are very central to the health of our society. You will cure. You will prophesy. You will guide our society in its most fundamental decisions.' Contrast this with what a person exhibiting schizophrenic activity in our society is told." [36]

The most conspicuous difference between the two approaches is the degree of shame heaped upon the heads of those with mental illness in our society. In the West, we fear madness and condemn to institutions and medication those who don't conform to our accepted norms. Branded, drugged and locked away, people in institutions are isolated and treated as problems so it is no wonder that their expectations and experience would be entirely negative. Without the support of culture, community and connection, the schizophrenic feels marginalized, untouchable and abnormal. They don't fit in. As McKenna pointed out, it is the typical treatment of schizophrenia that "makes it incurable."

He goes on to say that "The world is not an unsolved problem for scientists or sociologists. The world is a living mystery: our birth, our death, our being in the moment

[36] http://www.wilderutopia.com/performance/literary/terence-mckenna-on-shaman-ic-schizophrenia-and-cultural-healing/

– these are mysteries. They are doorways opening on to unimaginable vistas of self-exploration, empowerment and hope for the human enterprise. And our culture has killed that, taken it away from us, made us consumers of shoddy products and shoddier ideals."

In his book, *Shamans Among Us*, psychiatrist Joseph Polimeni tells us that out of all the most pressing psychiatric problems "schizophrenia is in some ways, the most mysterious." He calls it "one of the greatest scientific enigmas" and goes on to say, "Despite a hundred years of study, there is still no cohesive understanding of the anatomical, physiological and psychological workings underlying schizophrenia. The very complexity of schizophrenia could be a sufficient explanation for its incomprehensibility. On the other hand, when a scientific problem is so intractable, one wonders about the inadvertent propagation of an unsuspected error."

Does any of this sound familiar? It took a paradigm shift in line with that required for quantum mechanics for researchers to come up with a shamanistic theory of schizophrenia that uses an evolutionary lens. This theory helps explain the "schizophrenia paradox" which puzzled researchers.

If the condition was genetic but prevented those afflicted from reproducing, how come it did not simply die out? As schizophrenia occurs universally in industrialized and remote populations alike with a steady incidence rate of about 1% (considered to be a high-prevalence condition in evolutionary terms) and appears to have been around for a very long time, something wasn't adding up. For schizophrenia to have endured, there must have been some sort of benefit attached to it for the hunter gatherer societies.

Enter the shaman or medicine man, also universal across all cultures. Shamanism is "humanity's most ancient spiritual, religious, and healing practice" [37]. So says Michael Winkelman, former associate professor in the School of Human Evolution and Social Change at Arizona State University. Shamanistic rituals date back to human prehistory and share many features across cultures, like altered states of consciousness, and visionary and supernatural experiences for healing.

In his book, Polimeni points out the remarkable similarities between shamanism and the 'disease' of schizophrenia. Globally, schizophrenia affects about 1% of the population. In societies that recognize shamans today, there are about one per 60-150 people or roughly 1%. Most shamans are male as are most schizophrenics. Shamans, like schizophrenics, are convinced they can perform magic. They both hear voices, have visions and out of body experiences (astral travel). Schizophrenics are generally diagnosed in their late teens to early twenties, the same time frame that shamans are recognized and begin training.

---

[37] https://anthropology.ua.edu/blogs/primatereligion/2014/04/14/shamanism/

The Cult of the Individual

> *"We have created a Star Wars civilization, with Stone Age emotions" ~ Edward Wilson*

Schizophrenics have dysregulation in certain areas of the brain that are responsible for helping us construct a sense of self. One particular structure, the temporo-parietal junction, or TPJ, is affected. The TPJ is important for what is called theory of mind or your ability to know where you end and other people begin and gives you an idea of where you are located physically in space and time. The right TPJ is specialized in thinking about other people's thoughts and is not involved in any other kind of logic.

Schizophrenics have trouble with all of these things that help the rest of us maintain and understand our separateness from others. Their self-perception dissolves and their "me" disappears. They lose their "normal sense of self as a feeling of unitary entity, the "I", that owns and authors its thoughts, emotions, body and actions." [38] One patient described it as feeling like she did not belong to herself anymore. [39]

Another way to describe this loss is a disintegration of the ego, exactly what happens to us in dreams. In spiritual

---

[38] http://www.schres-journal.com/article/S0920-9964(13)00371-X/fulltext
[39] https://www.ncbi.nlm.nih.gov/pmc/articles/PMC3661330/

terms, this is called an ego death, which is a type of spiritual growing pain but it happens when you are awake as in schizophrenia. Whichever way this death occurs, involuntarily through schizophrenia or voluntarily through a spiritual quest, it can be extremely unpleasant, frightening and confusing.

James Stewart is quoted as defining ego death as: "Simply put, it is the dying of the sense of self, of individuality, or of that which I conceive myself to be as perhaps different than what I am...the dying of the conceptualized sense of self. In many ways ego death at its optimum is the fluid flexibility of adjustment to the ongoing expansion into the mystery of consciousness, and at its most challenging, the horrifying experience of attachment and rigidity." [40]

As a schizophrenic, if you lived in an individualist culture and experienced an ego death, you would feel like a social pariah and willingly take drugs to make it all go away. If however, you lived in a collectivist culture, where the separation of the individual from society is less defined, you would feel less threatened and more contained. If that society included shamans, they would usher you through the crisis and help you reintegrate yourself. Either way, it would still be a crisis but in the individualist culture, it would be a negative one from which you might not recover.

---

[40] http://www.maps.org/news-letters/v20n1/v20n1-40to41.pdf

Schizophrenics tend to display reduced latent inhibition and are predisposed to psychosis. Latent inhibition is the ability to block out external stimuli but the schizophrenic has a thin veil where others have a wall. As the vast majority of brain activity is unconscious, being able to pick up more subconscious information from the environment allows schizophrenics to make connections that don't enter the awareness of neurotypicals. They have a flood of information that can be overwhelming but at the same time can give rise to creativity because of the potential for random and novel associations.

"Creative people, like those with psychotic illnesses, tend to see the world differently to most. It's like looking at a shattered mirror." ~ Mark Millard, UK psychologist [41]

What some people see as a mental disorder might just be a complete disregard for the rules or an inability to follow them because that someone is moving to the beat of a different drum. This is what creativity is all about—thinking outside of the proverbial box and being able to suspend disbelief. Being open to a wider range of possibilities and being able to see what others can't is part of genius.

We have all heard the supposed links between genius and madness, creativity and mental illness. Turns out it is

---

[41] http://www.bbc.com/news/10154775

simply not true, although the relatives of schizophrenics have been shown to score disproportionately high in creative careers. The cultural belief in the tortured genius however, just won't go away. John Nash, genius mathematician and Nobel laureate was a schizophrenic made famous by the movie *A Beautiful Mind*. There is speculation that Van Gogh was either bipolar, schizophrenic or borderline.

We are left to ponder if the environment is the deciding factor in whether a person is a creative genius because of their 'madness' or despite it. Treating schizophrenics as outcasts is a double whammy for them because of their lack of filters. Heaping shame on their heads and doping them with drugs would surely snuff out the creative spark before it had a chance to fully blossom. "[C]reative people tend to be more sensitive to the emotional environment around them and are less robust in withstanding hostility, intolerance or criticism. Indeed, the higher the level of emotional criticism within the family context, the higher the rate of schizophrenic and depressive relapses. When people go into a psychotic REM trance due to emotional arousal any criticism may well be acting like a post-hypnotic suggestion, compounding the condition." [42]

---

[42] http://www.bmj.com/rapid-response/2011/11/01/schizophrenia-waking-reality-processed-through-dreaming-brain

> *"People who hear voices and see things that aren't there can be classified into two groups. The first group are people who cannot cope with such phenomena. They are referred to as 'mentally ill.' The second group can cope with them and they are referred to as 'psychics.'"* [43]

Lucid Dreaming

Dreams have been described as an 'epiphenomenon' which means they are more of an accidental by-product of brain activity and not the main event. Others think that they do have a primary purpose and that is to prepare us for threats in the waking environment. Most of our emotions in dreams seem to be of the negative kind, like anger and anxiety, so we get to act out and practice different scenarios that presumably help us deal with them in real life. People with scary dreams are better equipped to deal with scary stuff in their waking lives.

Another way of looking at dreams is that they allow us to process negative emotions in a way that we can't or don't in the waking state where our egos can get in the way and cloud our judgement.

---

43 http://www.near-death.com/experiences/triggers/psychosis.html

> *"Unfortunately, in this culture, with few exceptions, we are not taught to dream."* ~ *Stephen LaBerge, Ph.D.*

Dreams are expanded consciousness. They are not an experience of intellect but of awareness. The drop is part of the ocean but it is also the whole ocean. "Tat Tvam Asi" = "I am that" from the Advaita Vedanta school of Vedic philosophy. All things are connected and we are not separate from each other or from anything. The dream and the dreamer are one.

A little over a century ago, Sigmund Freud wrote, "[T]he interpretation of dreams is the via regia (royal road) to a knowledge of the unconscious element in our psychic life." Whilst much of what Freud taught has fallen out of fashion in the past hundred years, this particular line of thought is back in style, especially with regard to lucid dreaming.

A lucid dreamer is one who is aware that they are in a dream. Just as there are degrees of sleep, there are degrees of wakefulness but lucid dreamers learn to be in both worlds at the same time and be awake in their dreams. They know that the dreams are their own creations and can direct them anywhere.

Lucid dreamers cannot help but become conscious of the enormous power of their imagination to do and be anything, and go anywhere. It is not so much about consciously influencing the dream as it is about becoming more aware of being limitless. Whilst the ability to fly to Mars or shapeshift is undeniably cool, it's not really the point but knowing you have that ability is. So lucid dreaming is a way to tap the deepest reserves of your identity as an unbounded spirit with powers to transform reality. Which reality? All of them. Maybe Rubin Naiman is right when he says that sleep is our "default state" because in sleep we have dreams and if we learn how to be lucid in those dreams, we can be whatever we want to be.

In his book *The Quantum Revelation: A Modern-Day Spiritual Treasure,* Paul Levy mentions a conversation a friend of his had with David Bohm (one of the most influential theoretical physicists of the 20th century) about doing physics experiments in lucid dreams. Bohm was excited about the idea and admitted he had occasionally done it too, confiding that he believed "lucid dreaming very likely held an important key to a deeper understanding of the connection between consciousness and the manifestation of our experience in the world—in both our night and waking dream-worlds."

Levy goes on to write, "The idea is to not just do physics experiments in our lucid dreams, but to recognize that life itself is potentially the dream within which we can become lucid. The more we recognize the dreamlike nature of our waking experience, the more our waking life will reflect back this realization and manifest itself in a dreamlike way, thereby increasing our lucidity even further. In a positive feedback loop, our ever-increasing lucidity, driven by consciousness, builds on itself and at a certain point becomes self-generating, reminiscent of Wheeler's idea of the universe as a self-excited circuit. Adding lucidity to our experience of life is a powerful spiritual practice, a form of 'dream yoga.' Becoming lucid in our waking dream changes everything." [44]

Hypnagogic naps

Hypnagogia refers to the twilight zone between wakefulness and sleep. It is referred to as the threshold consciousness and includes things like lucid dreaming and hallucinations. A hypnagogic nap is a split second nap where the intuition and insight from dreamland can be accessed deliberately.

Salvador Dali used these micro naps that lasted for less than a second and called them "slumber with a key." He would sit in a chair holding a metal key between his thumb and forefinger. On the floor, beneath the key, he would have a plate. As soon as he drifted off to sleep, the key would fall from his fingers and hit the plate, waking him up.

"The most characteristic slumber, the one most appropriate to the exercise of the art of painting...is

---

[44] http://www.awakeninthedream.com/lucid-dreaming-quantum-physics/

the slumber which I call 'the slumber with a key,' ... you must resolve the problem of 'sleeping without sleeping,' which is the essence of the dialectics of the dream, since it is a repose which walks in equilibrium on the taut and invisible wire which separates sleeping from waking." ~ Salvador Dali, *50 Secrets of Magic Craftsmanship*

He credited these flash naps for his artistic inspiration and used them in preparation for an afternoon of painting. He believed they refreshed him on every level. In that impossibly short space of time between sleep and wakefulness, the mind is in the hypnagogic state of consciousness, similar to that of REM sleep. Here anything is possible and everything is connected and for a brief moment you can dip into the world of your dreams and pull out insights.

You can experience this altered state of consciousness while fully awake and use it to solve problems or get new ideas. It has been called a form of dream catching and is possibly as right brained as you can get because you are in such a fluid and suggestible frame of mind, if only very briefly.

Dali claimed he learnt this technique from Capuchin monks. Other artists used it as did Beethoven, Einstein, Richard Wagner, Walter Scott, Nikola Tesla, Isaac Newton and Edison. Edison liked to sit with a steel ball bearing held lightly in each hand. As soon as he fell asleep, one of the balls would fall out of his hand and wake him.

And so, good night...

We hope you have enjoyed this little journey into the fascinating and mysterious world of sleep and that it has opened you up to the possibility of many worlds beyond. If it has caused a bit of a sea change in the way you observe reality, our dreams have come true.

Index

B

brain 16,
23, 26, 27, 28, 30,
31, 32, 33, 34, 35,
36, 37, 38, 41, 46,
64, 65, 68, 92, 101,
102, 106, 108, 109,
110, 114

brain waves 23,
31, 33

C

cancer 16,
17, 20, 21, 53, 102

consciousness
23, 24, 30, 87, 97,
99, 107, 111, 112,
113, 114

D

dementia 16,
20, 21, 34, 37

depression 20,
21, 51, 61, 82,

diabetes 16,
20, 21, 41

H

heart disease 16,
20, 21

I

immunity 25,
39

inflammation 17,
21, 51, 60, 62

O

obesity 20,
21, 62, 84

R

relationships 17,
20, 65

S

sleep 11,
15-21, 23-50, 52,
54, 55, 57-70

sleep deprivation
19, 21, 40

sleep-deprived
20

spiritual 20,
26, 92, 94, 96, 105,
106, 107, 112, 113

Want to travel deeper into the mysterious world of sleep and dreams? Need to order more copies for your enterprise? Please visit us at

TheHealingPowerOfSleep.com